The Anterior Approach for Hip Reconstruction

Guest Editor

PAUL E. BEAULÉ, MD, FRCSC

ORTHOPEDIC CLINICS OF NORTH AMERICA

www.orthopedic.theclinics.com

July 2009 • Volume 40 • Number 3

SAUNDERS an imprint of ELSEVIER, Inc.

W.B. SAUNDERS COMPANY
A Division of Elsevier Inc.

1600 John F. Kennedy Blvd. • Suite 1800 • Philadelphia, PA 19103-2899.

http://www.orthopedic.theclinics.com

ORTHOPEDIC CLINICS OF NORTH AMERICA Volume 40, Number 3
July 2009 ISSN 0030-5898, ISBN-10: 1-4377-1252-5, ISBN-13: 978-1-4377-1252-0

Editor: Debora Dellapena

Orthopedic Clinics of North America (ISSN 0030-5898) is published quarterly (For Post Office use only: Volume 40 issue 3 of 4) by Elsevier Inc., 360 Park Avenue South, New York, NY 10010-1710. Months of publication are January, April, July, and October. Business and Editorial Offices: 1600 John F. Kennedy Blvd., Suite 1800, Philadelphia, PA 19103-2899. Customer Service Office: 6277 Sea Harbor Drive, Orlando, FL 33887-4800. Periodicals postage paid at New York, NY and additional mailing offices. Subscription prices are $244.00 per year for (US individuals), $424.00 per year for (US institutions), $288.00 per year (Canadian individuals), $508.00 per year (Canadian institutions), $355.00 per year (international individuals), $508.00 per year (international institutions), $122.00 per year (US students), $177.00 per year (Canadian and international students). Foreign air speed delivery is included in all *Clinics* subscription prices. All prices are subject to change without notice. **POSTMASTER:** Send address changes to *Orthopedic Clinics of North America*, Elsevier Periodicals Customer Service, 11830 Westline Industrial Drive, St. Louis, MO 63146. Customer Service (orders, claims, online, change of address): Elsevier Periodicals Customer Service, 11830 Westline Industrial Drive, St. Louis, MO 63146. Tel: 1-800-654-2452 (U.S. and Canada); 314-453-7041 (outside U.S. and Canada). Fax: 314-453-5170. E-mail: journalscustomerservice-usa@elsevier.com (for print support); journalsonlinesupport-usa@elsevier.com (for online support).

Reprints. For copies of 100 or more, of articles in this publication, please contact the Commercial Reprints Department, Elsevier Inc., 360 Park Avenue South, New York, NY 10010-1710. Tel.: 212-633-3812; Fax: 212-462-1935; Email: reprints@elsevier.com.

Orthopedic Clinics of North America is covered in *MEDLINE/PubMed (Index Medicus), Cinahl, Excerpta Medica,* and *Cumulative Index to Nursing and Allied Health Literature.*

Printed and bound by CPI Group (UK) Ltd, Croydon, CR0 4YY

Transferred to Digital Print 2011

Contributors

GUEST EDITOR

PAUL E. BEAULÉ, MD, FRCSC
Head, Adult Reconstruction, The Ottawa
Hospital, University of Ottawa; Associate
Professor, University of Ottawa, Ottawa,
Ontario, Canada

AUTHORS

ANDREW F. AJLUNI, DO
Fellow, Joint Implant Surgeons, Inc.,
New Albany, Ohio

KAMALJEET BANGA, MD, DNB(Ortho)
Adult Reconstruction Unit, The Ottawa
Hospital, University of Ottawa, Ottawa,
Ontario, Canada

**CEFIN BARTON, MB, BCh, MRCS(Ed),
FRCS (Tr&Orth)**
Adult Reconstruction Unit, The Ottawa
Hospital, University of Ottawa, Ottawa,
Ontario, Canada

PAUL E. BEAULÉ, MD, FRCSC
Head, Adult Reconstruction, The Ottawa
Hospital, University of Ottawa; Associate
Professor, University of Ottawa, Ottawa,
Ontario, Canada

MÉLANIE L. BEAULIEU, MSc
Research Associate, School of Human
Kinetics, University of Ottawa, Ottawa, Ontario,
Canada

BENJAMIN BENDER, MD
Department of Orthopaedic Surgery,
Rothman Institute of Orthopaedics, Thomas
Jefferson University Hospital, Philadelphia,
Pennsylvania

BENOIT BENOIT, MD, FRCSC
Professeur Adjoint, Chirurgien orthopédique,
Hôpital Sacré-Coeur de Montréal, Université
de Montréal, Canada

KEITH R. BEREND, MD
Associate, Joint Implant Surgeons, Inc.; Mount
Carmel Health System, New Albany; Clinical
Assistant Professor, Department
of Orthopaedics, The Ohio State University,
Columbus, Ohio

MOHIT BHANDARI, MD, MSc, FRCSC
Division of Orthopedic Surgery, Department
of Surgery and Department of Clinical
Epidemiology and Biostatistics; McMaster
University, Member of The Anterior Total Hip
Arthroplasty Collaborative (ATHAC)
Investigators, Ontario, Canada

MARIO BIZZINI, MS, PT
Neuromuscular Research Laboratory,
Schulthess Clinic, Zurich, Switzerland

ALAN CHAPUT, PharmD, MD, MSc, FRCPC
Assistant Professor, Department
of Anesthesiology, The Ottawa Hospital,
University of Ottawa, Ottawa, Ontario, Canada

EDWARD T. CROSBY, MD, FRCPC
Professor, Department of Anesthesiology,
The Ottawa Hospital, University of Ottawa,
Ottawa, Ontario, Canada

HOLLY EVANS, MD, FRCPC
Assistant Professor, Department of
Anesthesiology, The Ottawa Hospital,
University of Ottawa, Ottawa, Ontario, Canada

WADE GOFTON, MD, MEd, FRCSC
Adult Reconstruction Service, The Ottawa
Hospital, University of Ottawa, Ottawa,
Ontario, Canada

WILLIAM J. HOZACK, MD
Professor, Department of Orthopaedic
Surgery, Rothman Institute of Orthopaedics,
Thomas Jefferson University Hospital,
Philadelphia, Pennsylvania

FRANCO M. IMPELLIZZERI, MS
Neuromuscular Research Laboratory,
Schulthess Clinic, Zurich, Switzerland

MICHAEL S.H. KAIN, MD
Fellow, M.E. Müller Foundation North America;
Schulthess Clinic, Zurich, Switzerland

CHRISTOPHER KIM, MSc
Department of Surgery, Division of
Orthopedics, The Ottawa Hospital, University
of Ottawa, Ottawa, Ontario, Canada

PAUL R. KIM, MD, FRCSC
Division of Orthopedics, Adult Reconstruction
Unit, The Ottawa Hospital, University
of Ottawa, Ottawa, Ontario, Canada

MARIO LAMONTAGNE, PhD
Full Professor, School of Human Kinetics;
Department of Mechanical Engineering,
University of Ottawa, Ottawa, Ontario, Canada

ALAN LANE, MB, FCARCSI
Assistant Professor, Department of
Anesthesiology, The Ottawa Hospital,
University of Ottawa, Ottawa, Ontario, Canada

ALEJANDRO LAZO-LANGNER, MD, MSc
Assistant Professor, Departments of Medicine
and Oncology, University of Western Ontario;
London Health Sciences Centre, Victoria
Hospital, London, Ontario, Canada

MICHAEL LEUNIG, MD
Associate Professor, Department
of Orthopedic Surgery, University Bern;
Consultant, Schulthess Clinik, Zurich,
Switzerland

ADOLPH V. LOMBARDI, Jr., MD, FACS
President, Joint Implant Surgeons, Inc.; Mount
Carmel Health System, New Albany; Clinical
Assistant Professor, Departments of
Orthopaedics and Biomedical Engineering,
The Ohio State University, Columbus, Ohio

NICOLA A. MAFFIULETTI, PhD
Neuromuscular Research Laboratory,
Schulthess Clinic, Zurich, Switzerland

NICHOLAS H. MAST, MD
The Hip and Pelvis Institute, St. John's Health
Center, Santa Monica, California

JOEL MATTA, MD
The Hip and Pelvis Institute, St. John's Health
Center, Santa Monica, California

HIDENOBU MIKI, MD
Department of Orthopedic Surgery, National
Hospital Organization Osaka National Hospital,
Osaka, Japan

MICHELLE MUÑOZ, BA
The Hip and Pelvis Institute, St. John's Health
Center, Santa Monica, California

URS MUNZINGER, MD
Lower Extremity Unit, Schulthess Clinic,
Zurich, Switzerland

NOBUO NAKAMURA, MD
Director, Center of Arthroplasty, Kyowakai
Hospital, Osaka, Japan

TAKASHI NISHII, MD
Associate Professor, Department of
Orthopedic Surgery, Osaka University
Graduate School of Medicine, Osaka, Japan

MICHAEL NOGLER, MD, MA, MAS, MSc
Professor; Vice Chairman of the Department
of Orthopaedic Surgery, Medical University
of Innsbruck, Innsbruck, Austria

FRANZ RACHBAUER, MD, MSc
Associate Professor, Department of
Orthopedic Surgery, Medical University;
Consultant, Department of Orthopedics,
Landeskrankenhaus, Innsbruck, Austria

MARC A. RODGER, MD, MSc, FRCPC
Associate Professor, Departments of Medicine
Epidemiology and Community Medicine, and
Obstetrics and Gynecology, University of
Ottawa; Deputy Director and Senior Scientist,
Clinical Epidemiology Program, Ottawa Health
Research Institute, Ottawa, Ontario, Canada

TAKASHI SAKAI, MD
Assistant Professor, Department of Orthopedic
Surgery, Osaka University Graduate School of
Medicine, Osaka, Japan

BRIAN E. SENG, DO
Fellow, Joint Implant Surgeons, Inc., New
Albany, Ohio

NOBUHIKO SUGANO, MD
Professor, Department of Orthopedic Surgery,
Osaka University Graduate School of
Medicine, Osaka, Japan

MASAKI TAKAO, MD
Department of Orthopedic Surgery, Osaka
University Graduate School of Medicine,
Osaka, Japan

RAYMOND TANG, MSc, MD, FRCPC
Fellow, Department of Anesthesiology, The
Ottawa Hospital, University of Ottawa, Ottawa,
Ontario, Canada

DANIEL VARIN, BSc
Research Assistant, School of Human Kinetics,
University of Ottawa, Ottawa, Ontario, Canada

KATHARINA WIDLER, MS
Neuromuscular Research Laboratory,
Schulthess Clinic, Zurich, Switzerland

Contents

The History of the Anterior Approach to the Hip　　　　　　　　　　**311**

Franz Rachbauer, Michael S.H. Kain, and Michael Leunig

> The anterior approach is a safe, reliable, and feasible technique for total hip arthro-plasty, permitting optimal soft tissue preservation. Since Hueter first described this interval, many surgeons have approached the hip anteriorly to perform a myriad of surgical procedures. The anterior approach allows optimal muscle preservation, and it is a truly internervous approach to the hip. An understanding of the evolution of the anterior approach to the hip will help the orthopedic community understand these advantages and why so many have used this approach in the treatment of hip pathology and for the implantation total hip arthroplasty.

Direct Anterior Approach for Total Hip Arthroplasty　　　　　　　　**321**

Benjamin Bender, Michael Nogler, and William J. Hozack

> This article describes the surgical technique for total hip arthroplasty using the single-incision direct anterior approach. The authors believe the direct anterior approach has significant advantages, including minimal soft tissue trauma, resulting in faster postoperative mobilization and rehabilitation. The small incision scar also results in better cosmesis.

Outcomes Following the Single-Incision Anterior Approach to Total Hip Arthroplasty: A Multicenter Observational Study　　　　　　　　　　　　　　　　　　**329**

The Anterior Total Hip Arthroplasty Collaborative (ATHAC) Investigators

> The authors conducted a retrospective, multicenter cohort study of 1,152 patients across nine clinical sites across the United States, evaluating complications and function associated with the anterior approach to total hip arthroplasty using an or-thopedic table. Eligible patients included those with primary diagnosis of hip arthri-tis. Outcomes included hospital stay, use of assistive devices, complications, and function. In the cohort of 1,152 patients treated with the anterior approach to total hip arthroplasty, the authors found (*i*) an acceptable complication profile with a very low dislocation rate, (*ii*) an early return to function, and (*iii*) a decline in com-plications in surgeons with greater than 100 case experiences.

Anterior-Supine Minimally Invasive Total Hip Arthroplasty: Defining the Learning Curve　　　　　　　　　　　　　　　　　　　　　　　　　**343**

Brian E. Seng, Keith R. Berend, Andrew F. Ajluni, and Adolph V. Lombardi, Jr.

> The anterior-supine intermuscular approach is a truly muscle-sparing approach to to-tal hip arthroplasty with a low complication rate. The advantages include improved early recovery and return to everyday activities. The authors found the learning curve to be around 40 cases and 6 months in a high-volume joint surgeon's practice. This article provides a detailed description of the surgical approach, including the use of a standard operating room table and fluoroscopy. Cadaver dissections and one-on-one mentoring are recommended when implementing this approach in one's practice.

Multimodal analgesia incorporates the use of analgesic adjuncts with different mechanisms of action to enhance postoperative pain management. Acetaminophen, anti-inflammatories, and gabapentinoids provide effective analgesia while reducing opioid requirements and opioid-related side effects. Intrathecal morphine and periarticular local anesthetic infiltration further enhance dynamic analgesia and improve postoperative mobilization. Epidural analgesia, peripheral nerve blocks, tramadol, ketamine, and/or clonidine can be added for improved benefit in opioid-tolerant individuals.

In the last decade, femoro–acetabular impingement (FAI) has been recognized as a cause of pain and early arthrosis in the young adult hip. Carl Hueter first described the anterior approach in 1881. This article discusses the indications and diagnostic criteria and the surgical technique and early clinical results for the combined arthroscopic/Hueter approach.

This article presents critical issues related to the interpretation of biomechanical findings of the hip joint for patients having undergone hip arthroplasty. The use of a gait, or biomechanical, analysis provides objective evidence of the efficiency of the treatments or the effectiveness of hip replacement approaches. Based on our biomechanical analysis, patients who have undergone total hip arthroplasty use a stair ascent and descent strategy allowing them to significantly reduce loading at the prosthetic hip joint. Since hip joint reaction forces are highly dependent on muscle activation, the THA group have adopted a neuromuscular control strategy that is enabling them to reduce loading on the prosthetic hip joint. It could also be a joint loading pattern that stems from a muscular deficiency emerging either from several years of loading avoidance on the affected hip joint or from the surgical procedure. Therefore, a biomechanical analysis of human motion is a valuable tool for the orthopedic surgeon to objectively quantify joint motion and the forces producing this motion.

The objective of this preliminary study was to examine possible differences in gait characteristics between subjects operated by way of a direct anterior approach and a posterior approach for primary total-hip arthroplasty, and age-matched healthy controls. Fifty-one subjects walked over an instrumented mat at two different speeds (self-selected comfortable and faster than normal) and spatiotemporal gait parameters were calculated using a validated methodology. Despite excellent clinical and radiographic scores, and irrespective of surgical approach, patients demonstrated an impaired walking performance (lower velocity and shorter step lengths) during fast walking, but not at the self-selected comfortable speed compared with healthy controls. Subjects operated with the posterior approach reported significantly higher stiffness than anterior subjects, but similar pain and function. Six months after total arthroplasty for primary osteoarthritis of the hip, gait characteristics were comparable between subjects having received the direct anterior approach and the posterior approach.

Blood conservation techniques are well established and have significant benefits. We review the current literature on these techniques and their applicability to hip reconstruction surgery and offer a suitable strategy to minimize allogeneic red cell transfusion.

Venous thromboembolic disease continues to be a serious complication of total-hip arthroplasty. The use of anticoagulant drugs for preventing this complication has repeatedly been proven to be useful. This article reviews the current evidence-based recommendations for anticoagulant prophylaxis after total-hip arthroplasty and provides insight into the current areas of active research and controversy.

Orthopedic Clinics of North America

THE CLINICS ARE NOW AVAILABLE ONLINE!

Access your subscription at:
www.theclinics.com

Orthopedic Clinics of North America

Preface

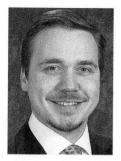

Paul E. Beaulé, MD, FRCSC
Guest Editor

The practice of hip surgery has evolved tremendously in the last decade. We have witnessed the introduction of less invasive surgical techniques, rapid recovery programs, and a better understanding of the cause of idiopathic hip arthritis within the concept of femoroacetabular impingement. As we continue to explore and improve the management of hip pathology, patients also want to maintain a high activity level and minimize their recovery time after undergoing reconstructive hip surgery.

Thus, it is quite appropriate that the anterior approach to the hip joint classically known as Smith Peterson but initially described by a German surgeon, Carl Hueter, is being more widely used and applied to the field of hip surgery. More importantly, the anterior approach is the only approach to the hip that is purely inter-nervous and intermuscular while providing adequate access to perform a variety of reconstructive hip procedures regardless of the patient's body habitus. Because of the limited soft tissue dissection associated with this approach, an optimal rehabilitation environment is provided to the patient without compromising the correction of the underlying surgical pathology. The versatility of the anterior approach and the advantages of having the patient in the supine position is well illustrated in this issue of *Orthopaedic Clinics of North America,* which, once again, is at the forefront of new advances in orthopaedic surgery. The clinical research presented in this issue from various authors illustrates the large clinical experience with the anterior approach, as well as its safety and efficacy in performing primary hip replacements, hip resurfacing, and impingement surgery. In addition, this issue discusses the capacity of using three-dimensional motion analysis to better understand hip kinematics, as well as improve our understanding of the clinical impact of the different surgical approaches on patient function after hip replacement surgery. Finally, two review articles present the latest in multi-modal anesthesia and thrombophylaxis, further optimizing the return to normal function of our patients.

As Guest Editor and user of the anterior approach, being able to demonstrate that the anterior approach can provide reproducible results from a variety of centers with a relatively low complication rate is a key element for the widespread use of any surgical technique. It has been a great honor to have had the opportunity to serve as a Guest Editor of this issue of *Orthopaedic Clinics of North America,* and I would like to thank all the authors who took the time to contribute their scientific work to this issue, as well as Deb Dellapena for her assistance.

Paul E. Beaulé, MD, FRCSC
Adult Reconstruction, The Ottawa Hospital
University of Ottawa
501 Smyth Road CCW 1646
Ottawa, Ontario, Canada

E-mail address:
pbeaule@ottawahospital.on.ca (P.E. Beaulé)

Orthop Clin N Am 40 (2009) xiii
doi:10.1016/j.ocl.2009.06.001

orthopedic.theclinics.com

The History of the Anterior Approach to the Hip

Franz Rachbauer, MD, MSc[a],*, Michael S.H. Kain, MD[b,c],
Michael Leunig, MD[c]

KEYWORDS

- Hip • Anterior approach • History
- Minimally invasive • Anatomy

No, 'tis not so deep as a well,
nor so wide as a church-door;
but 'tis enough, 'twill serve.
(Shakespeare, Romeo and Juliet)

The anterior approach to the hip takes advantage of the interval between the sartorius muscle and the tensor fascia lata muscle to access the hip joint. The upper aspect of this approach provides visualization of and access to the entire ileum and hip joint. Nearly all surgery of the hip can be performed through this approach or through different portions of the approach. The anterior approach remains a standard approach to the hip in pediatric orthopedic surgery for developmental hip dysplasia, whereas in adult orthopedic surgery it is used mostly to expose the anterolateral aspect of the femoral head, the femoral neck, and the anterior aspect of the acetabulum to treat femoral head fractures, for biopsy, or for excision of ectopic bone.[1] With increasing interest in femoroacetabular impingement, hip resurfacing, and minimally invasive total hip arthroplasty, the anterior approach has regained popularity as a versatile approach to the hip in adult orthopedic patients. To refocus the knowledge about and interest in the anterior approach, a foray into its history might be useful.

DEFINITION

Surgical approaches are anatomic dissections of tissue planes that use anatomic knowledge to limit the amount of dissection required to perform the procedure while avoiding nerve and vessel damage.[1] Anatomically, the hip can be approached from various directions—posterior, anterolateral, lateral, lateral transtrochanteric, medial, or anterior—and each approach has advantages and disadvantages. These various approaches to the hip are associated with many eponyms, usually a tribute to the originating surgeon. This article focuses on the anterior approach to the hip joint, as defined by the interval between the sartorius and tensor fasciae latae, commonly referred to as the "Smith-Petersen approach" or the "Hueter approach."[1]

HISTORY

Published accounts do not necessarily describe all the original attempts and successes of a surgical technique. Fully aware of these limitations, the authors have made a sincere attempt to obtain the original written sources and to interpret them correctly. They apologize if any significant contributions were misunderstood or neglected; no disrespect is intended.

[a] Department of Orthopedic Surgery, Landeskrankenhaus/Medical University Innsbruck, Anichstrasse 35, A-6020 Innsbruck, Austria
[b] M.E. Müller Foundation North America, 69A Dartmouth Street #2, Belmont, MA 02478, USA
[c] Schulthess Clinik, Lengghalde 2, CH-8008, Zurich, Switzerland
* Corresponding author. Department of Orthopedic Surgery, Medical University Innsbruck, Anichstrasse 35, A-6020 Innsbruck, Austria.
E-mail address: Franz.rachbauer@i-med.ac.at (F. Rachbauer).

Orthop Clin N Am 40 (2009) 311–320
doi:10.1016/j.ocl.2009.02.007

The first written description of the anterior approach to the hip might be attributed to Carl Hueter, a German surgeon, author of several medical articles and books, and a member of the German Imperial Diet.[2] Hueter was born in Marburg, on November 27, 1838, where his father, Karl Christoph Hueter, served as professor of surgery and gynecology. He began studying medicine in 1854, at the age of 16 years, and was promoted to medical doctor in 1858, while in Kassel, following educational journeys to Vienna, Berlin, England, and Scotland. Hueter later worked at the Anatomic Institute in Paris from 1861 to 1863, studying human joints. He went on to serve as an assistant to Virchow and later Langenbeck before obtaining academic accreditation in 1868.[3] Other surgeons, such as Bernhard Bardenheuer (1839–1913), Otto Gerhard Karl Sprengel (1852–1915), and Larghi, have been mentioned as possible originators of the anterior approach, but Hueter's classic work, *Der Grundriss der Chirurgie* (*The Compendium of Surgery*), published in 1881 (**Fig. 1**), is the first to describe the anterior approach to the hip[4,5] as used today:

The anterior oblique incision for resectio coxae was first performed by Lücke and then by Max Schede. I have adopted this incision with a modification that I will explain later on. Following numerous experiences in the living and dead I have established the method as follows.

*Define the anterior iliac spine and the tip of the greater trochanter. Halve the line between the two points and pierce the tip of the knife in the middle of this line with the blade directed caudally and somewhat inferiorly. The incision is directed parallel to the outer border of the Sartorius muscle (see **Fig. 1**), but somewhat external; in children 6–8 cm, in adults relative to muscular development 10–15 cm. It falls into the muscular interstice between m. sartorius on one side and m. tensor fasciae latae and m. gluteus medius on the other side, and meets the fibers of the m. vastus lateralis, which originate at the anterior face of the trochanter major at the base of the femoral neck. Those fibers have to be detached by knife or elevator; but it is the only muscle which is injured through the operation; and only in a small part of its fibers. Knife and elevator pierce into the anterior face of the major trochanter and the femoral neck. At the lower border of the femoral neck preference has to be given to the elevator to prevent transection of the anterior circumflex artery.*

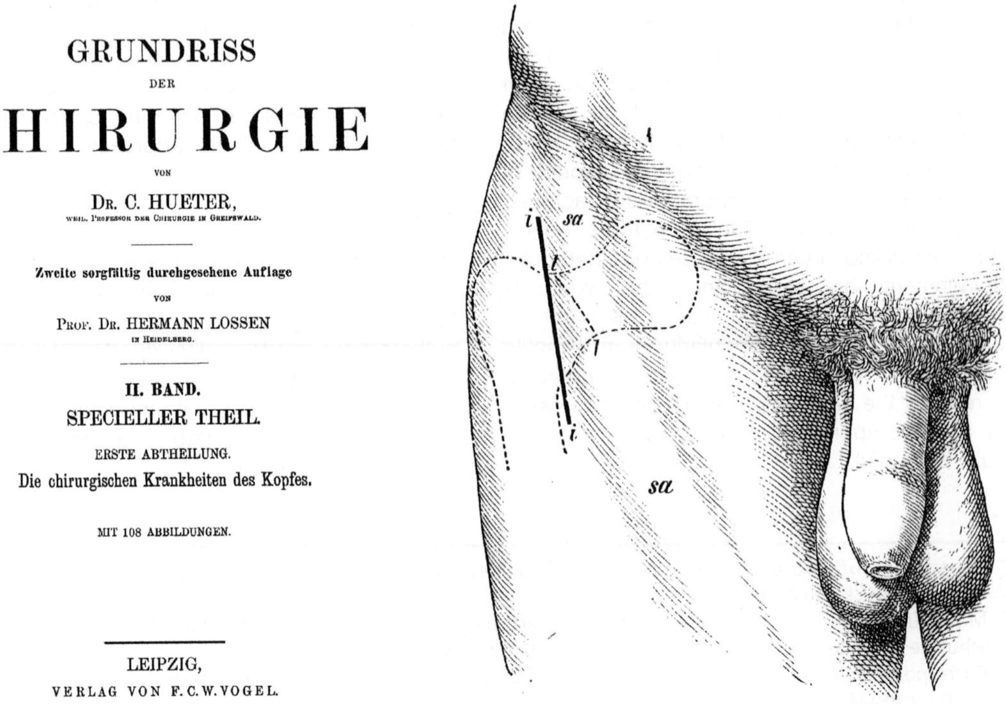

Fig. 1. Title page of "Grundriβ der Chirurgie" and the original drawing illustrating the approach. (*From* C. Hueter, Grundriss der Chirurgie, 2nd edition. Leipzig: FCW Vogel; 1883.)

Following the opening of the hip joint capsule, it is cut with the probe-pointed knife superiorly and inferiorly as much as possible; the femoral neck can be encompassed by the index finger superiorly and inferiorly within the capsule. ... The advantages of the anterior oblique approach are: (1) Only one muscle, the m. vastus ext. is injured; for this reason the leg keeps its tight connections to the pelvis which facilitates rehabilitation; (2) bleeding is so little, that no single ligature has to be done ...[4]

Marius N. Smith-Petersen (1886–1953), a Norwegian-born American surgeon,[1] is credited with spreading the use of the anterior approach in the English-speaking world, and today the approach is commonly referred to as the "Smith-Petersen approach" because of his prolific use of the approach throughout his career. In his Moynihan Lecture in 1947,[6] Smith-Petersen recounted his original planning and execution of the anterior approach to the hip joint in 1917 (**Fig. 2**):

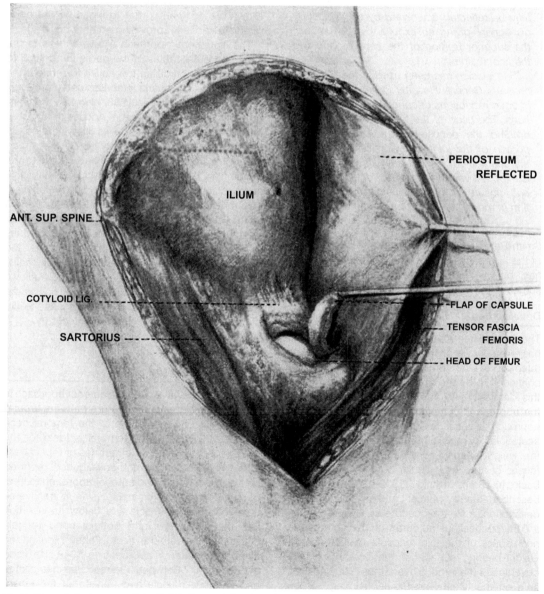

Fig. 2. The original approach by Smith-Petersen in 1917. (*From* MN Smith-Petersen. A new supra-articular subperiosteal approach to the hip joint. J Bone Joint Surg Am 1917;s2–15;595.)

In connection with hip-joint surgery at the Massachusetts General Hospital Orthopedic Clinic, an incision has suggested itself to the writer, which seems to offer promise of usefulness in certain types of operations. The commonly used anterior incision does not give a very good exposure of the acetabulum; this structure is found at the bottom of an abyss-like hole, sometimes only felt, and in still other cases the operator is uncertain whether the structure he feels is the acetabulum or the supra-articular notch. If, however, the usual anterior incision be extended backward from the anterior superior spine along the crest of the ilium, the flap thus formed may be reflected downward by subperiosteal dissection, giving an excellent exposure of the superior portion of the capsule and of the acetabulum. ...

This incision has been used in the Massachusetts General Hospital Orthopedic Clinic in open reductions of congenital hip dislocations. The head of the femur is exposed by dividing the periosteum and the superior portion of the joint capsule; it is placed in the acetabulum without any difficulty as this is exposed very well indeed. After reduction and closure of the capsule the hip is quite firm in moderate abduction.[7]

Following Hueter's original description and Smith-Petersen's continued use and development of the approach, the anterior approach to the hip has been used and re-described by many surgeons to treat various hip disorders.

Developmental Hip Dysplasia

The surgical treatment of developmental dysplasia has relied heavily on the Hueter interval, commonly referred to by Smith-Petersen himself, and continues to be the main approach used to treat this deformity. As in the original description of the approach, the extended anterior, iliofemoral approach is ideal for the surgical treatment of acetabular dysplasia. The technique of enlarging the weight-bearing zone of the acetabulum by means of an extra-articular bony extension goes back to Franz König (1832–1910) and was described later by Marcel Lance, in 1925.[8] In this description, a shelf procedure consisted of fitting a corticocancellous autograft on the anterosuperior aspect of the joint capsule to increase the weight-bearing surface of the acetabulum and coverage of the femoral head, thus reducing pressure on the healthy acetabular cartilage. In the 1960s, a number of authors (among them Judet and Roy-Camille) modified the original technique

to improve graft placement and graft fixation. These modifications continued to use an incision similar to the Smith-Petersen approach and the Hueter interval.[9]

In 1961 Salter[10] successfully used the anterior approach for his innominate osteotomy in the treatment of congenital dislocation and subluxation of the hip. For this procedure the approach provides access to the inner and outer tables of the pelvis, enabling the surgeon to osteotomize the ileum from the sciatic notch completely. Pemberton[11] also described a pericapsular osteotomy via a Smith-Peterson approach in 1965. His osteotomy, better suited for the younger patient with an open triradiate cartilage and dysplasia, allows the acetabular roof to hinge on the open triradiate cartilage, providing anterior coverage.

The iliofemoral approach allows access to the inner and outer tables of the pelvis in addition to the hip joint, optimizing the ability to reorient the acetabulum. The periacetabular osteotomy, as advocated by Ganz[12] in 1988, also takes advantage of the anterior approach. Access to the inner table in the true and false pelvis allows the polygonal, juxta-articular osteotomy to be performed while preserving the vascular blood supply to the acetabular fragment, thus allowing an extensive acetabular reorientation to improve insufficient coverage of the femoral head and for medialization of the joint. This technique allows the continued treatment of residual hip dysplasia in young adults to prevent secondary coxarthritis, even after the closure of the triradiate cartilage. Additionally, the modified Smith-Petersen approach allows a simultaneous anterior capsulotomy to visualize the hip joint and the labrum or to assess the hip dynamically before and after the osteotomy.

Fractures of the Hip

Many surgeons have used the anterior approach in the treatment of various fracture patterns around the hip. Direct visualization of the femoral neck and easy access to the femoral is ideal for the treatment of femoral neck fractures or Pipkin fractures. In 1939 Cubbins and colleagues[13] reported on the use of a modified anterior approach to treat fractures of the femur neck using a transverse transection of the fascia lata below its insertion into the fascia lata and iliotibial band to gain access to the femoral neck. Fahey[14] described a modified anterior approach in 1949. He used the interval between tensor fasciae latae and sartorius muscle and transected the tensor at the lower border of the incision. When necessary, the tensor fasciae latae and gluteus medius muscle were stripped subperiosteally from the iliac wing.

A few years later, in 1943, Levine[15] reported the successful treatment of a central fracture of the acetabulum via an anterior approach. More specifically Levine was the first to modify the Smith-Petersen approach to expose the inner table of the pelvis. The Judet brothers used the anterior approach frequently for arthroplasty procedure and later, in cooperation with Emile Letournel, used the approach for the treatment of pelvic fractures:

> Since 1954, we have paid particular attention to the study of fractures of the acetabulum. Because we were so disappointed with the results of closed treatment of these fractures, we decided to try open reduction. Our series included 173 patients of whom 129 were treated surgically … . To reach the anterior aspect of the acetabulum, we used an ileoc-rural approach. This approach extends along the anterior half of the crest of the ileum as far as the anterosuperior iliac spine and the runs obliquely anteriorly and medially along the lateral aspect of the sartorius muscle for about fifteen centimetres.[16]

Letournel then described an extension of the anterior iliofemoral approach for the treatment of acetabular fractures, that is, the extended iliofemoral approach:

> The incision is in form of an inverted J. Beginning at the posterior superior iliac spine, it follows the ileac crest as far as the anterior-superior iliac spine and from there descends straight toward the outer border of the patella half way down the thigh. … This approach includes the tensor fascia lata of which the anterior border is followed. The dissection remains in the fibrous sheath of the muscle to avoid, as far as possible, dividing the branches of the lateral cutaneous nerve of the thigh.[17]

The extended iliofemoral approach is still used today, but the indications for this extensile approach have decreased for many surgeons, who fear the morbidity associated with a devitalized gluteal flap secondary to injury to the superior gluteal artery. Nevertheless, a recent publication by Griffin and colleagues[18] has shown it to be safe and effective, with the major complication being heterotopic ossification.

This approach is not limited to use in fracture patients, because it is a well-known approach for type I and II hemipelvectomy in tumor surgery.[19]

Finally, with an increasing number of osteoporotic acetabular fractures being seen, Beaulé and colleagues[20] have described using the anterior approach to treat acetabular fractures with a total hip arthroplasty.

Femoro-Acetabular Impingement

In 1936 Smith-Petersen developed an acetabuloplasty operation through the anterior approach to relieve pain and restore function in what today might be considered osteoarthritis of the hip.[21] In this respect he anticipated the recent developments on femoroacetabular impingement surgery:

> A plastic procedure has been proposed for the relief of hip-joint conditions resulting from interference with the normal mechanics of the hip joint. Such conditions are "malum coxae senilis," "interapelvic protrusion of the acetabulum," "old slipped upper femoral epiphysis," "fractures of the the neck of the femur with malposition," "Legg-Calvé-Perthes disease," and "fractures of the acetabulum."[21]

As surgical treatment for femoral acetabular impingement evolves, surgeons are using a variety of approaches to improve the femoral neck offset. The originators describe the use of the surgical dislocation,[22] and others have relied on arthroscopy as the surgical approach.[23] The anterior approach has also gained attention as a surgical technique to for these patients. Clohisy and colleagues[24] described a combination of open surgery and arthroscopy in which a mini-anterior approach was used to perform the osteochondroplasty of the femoral head after the joint was evaluated with arthroscopy.

Other Arthritic Conditions

Patients who have osteonecrosis or avascular necrosis of the femoral head usually are doomed to total hip arthroplasty once the femoral head has collapsed. To prevent further damage to the femoral head and its collapse, Hisashi and colleagues[25] described the use of the anterior approach to access the femoral neck and head for bone grafting of the femoral head. The anterior approach is ideal for this technique, and the excellent access to the femoral neck and head allows a window to be made in the femoral neck so that nonvascularized and/or vascularized bone grafts can be introduced into the femoral neck and head after debridement of the necrotic bone:

> Surgery involved curettage of necrotic bone, implantation of spongy bone, and application

of a vascularized pedicle bone graft. Grafts were taken from the ileum and included the circumflex iliac artery. A bony canal was made in the anterior femoral neck, from which the necrotic bone was curetted and to which the bone graft was applied.[25]

When death of the femoral head was inevitable, arthrodesis was a more commonly accepted technique, and in 1950 Kirkaldy-Willis[26] described the ischiofemoral arthrodesis, consisting of bone grafting via the anterior approach for treatment of healed tuberculosis of the hip without gross destruction. Since then, in 1997, Matta and colleagues[27] also reported on a technique for hip fusion through the anterior approach with the use of a ventral plate.

The Evolution of Anterior Approach Arthroplasty

In addition to his work in the treatment of dysplasia, Smith-Petersen also focused on treating end-stage arthritis of the hip and developed a Vitallium-mold arthroplasty, after preliminary trials of several materials, including glass (1923), Viscoloid (1925), Pyrex (1933), and Bakelite (1938). He described his rationale for using the Hueter interval for such an implant:

A joint has two surfaces which must be so shaped as to be able to function without interference or impingement through the greatest possible arc. Consequently, in the case of the hip joint, it is necessary to expose the acetabulum and its adjacent structures, as well as the femoral head and neck. In the past the various approaches to the hip joint have failed to properly expose the acetabulum, and the surgeon's efforts have been directed mainly at partial reconstruction of the femoral head. Reconstruction of the acetabulum demands intrapelvic exposure of this side of the joint. The approach to such an exposure necessitates extensive dissection; since this can be performed along structural planes, it is not destructive.[28]

Continuing with this philosophy, the Judets[29] reported the use of the anterior approach for hip hemiarthroplasty in 1950, when they described a "resection-reconstruction" as being the

excision of the pathologic femoral head and its replacement by an artificial head, made of a synthetic plastic material, which is firmly fixed to the upper end of the femur. This study

is based on 300 cases, the earliest of which dates back some three and a half years. ... To obtain good movement later we believe that it is essential to avoid all damage to muscle and bone. We therefore use Hueter's vertical incision, which extends about 15 centimetres down from the anterior-superior iliac spine, passes between tensor fasciae latae and sartorius, then lateral to rectus femoris and down to the capsule.[29]

In 1955, O'Brien[30] from Saint Louis described the insertion of a femoral head prosthesis via the straight anterior approach: "Since November, 1951, we have employed the Fred Thomson prosthesis almost exclusively. ... Hueter's anterior straight incision, to be discussed here, does not require muscle cutting or detachment, and no postoperative immobilization is needed."[30]

At first the anterior approach was used to minimize muscle damage, but some surgeons found the approach limiting. While reporting on the insertion of a stemmed medullary femoral component using a modified anterior approach, Luck[31], from Los Angeles in 1955, described how the Hueter approach hindered the placement of such a prosthesis. The skepticism expressed by Luck lingered for years, and with Charnley's[32] reports of success using the transtrochanteric approach, the Hueter approach was used less frequently.

Surgeons interested in the development of the modern resurfacing techniques, such as Wagner,[33] saw significant advantages to using of the anterior approach. In 1978 Wagner described his rationale for using the anterior approach for resurfacing:

Although total joint replacement using any of the well tested variants of total prosthesis today, represents an effective means of operative correction in severe hip disability of many etiologies it has several inherent shortcomings. The major disadvantage result from the sacrifice of the femoral head and neck, so that should the prosthesis fail no completely satisfactory alternative exists. ... An anterior approach is used and considered the key to a successful procedure. For hip joint resurfacing in difficult cases the anterior approach is essential as it allows optimum exposure of both acetabulum and femoral head and neck, provides maximum soft tissue release, and allows preservation of the important posterior retinacular vessels. In addition the muscles are separated in the interspace between femur and gluteal innervation and vascularization which is important for wound healing and subsequent function.

Particularly in cases of severe deformity and/or contracture the anterior approach is the key to successful operation.[33]

As total hip arthroplasty continued to evolve, the Judets[34] again took up the baton. In 1985 they described the procedure of a total hip arthroplasty through an anterior approach with the assistance of an orthopedic table:

The anterior approach to the hip is first between the tensor muscle of fascia lata and the sartorius muscle, then laterally to the vastus externus. Deinsertion of the fascia lata from the ileum is necessary in only slightly more than one half of the cases, and it is always limited. Access to the capsule is wide and, provided one works on an orthopedic operating table, the maneuvers required to dislocate the joint and expose the femoral head and neck, then the cotyloid cavity, are simple. Closure is easy and because the trochanter has not been sectioned, early rehabilitation is possible.[34]

Light and Keggi[35] advocated the splitting of the tensor fasciae latae for straightforward, effective exposure for total hip arthroplasty, an approach they dubbed an "anterior approach for hip arthroplasty":

Our anterior approach employs a curved transverse or short straight skin incision with or without a small proximal incision, or stab wound, to allow for the precise passage of femoral reamers and prosthetic components, and occasionally an additional small distal incision for the passage of acetabular instruments. The primary skin incision is similar to the proximal incision of a Watson-Jones approach or the distal portion of a Smith-Peterson incision and allows exposure of the underlying tensor fasciae latae muscle. Slitting the anterior fibers of the tensor fascia latae easily exposes the anterior hip joint capsule.[35]

Recently they reported on using the split approach with the addition of a second and third incision in more than 2000 patients.[36] Other variations of the anterior approach have been reported also. In 2003 Berger[37] popularized the idea of minimally invasive total hip arthroplasty. His two-incision approach combines a small anterior approach for cup insertion and a second transgluteal incision for the insertion of the femoral implant. The failures of the technique in other hands cannot be blamed to the meticulously elaborated nailing technique developed by Kuentscher[38] that obviously served as a blueprint for the second incision site of Berger's technique.

With the advent of minimally invasive total hip arthroplasty, the anterior approach, as proposed by the brothers Judet[34] using an orthopedic traction table (**Fig. 3**), has gained popularity through the reports by Siguier and collegues[39] and Matta and colleagues.[40] Nevertheless, the need for using an orthopedic table seems to have hindered the technique's wider acceptance.

The authors and colleagues have started to investigate the use of an minimally invasive anterior approach for conventional total hip arthroplasty without the use of an orthopedic table (**Figs. 3–5**).[41–46]

Several studies have indicated that minimally invasive posterior, transgluteal, and anterolateral approaches have no significant advantages over more conventional approaches. This result might be anticipated, because the theoretical benefits

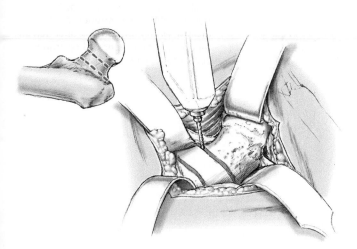

Fig. 3. In situ osteotomy of the femoral neck via an anterior approach for minimally invasive total hip arthroplasty. (*From* Rachbauer F, Krismer M. Minimal-invasive Hüftendoprothetik über den anterioren Zugang. Oper Orthop Traumatol 2008;20:245; with permission.)

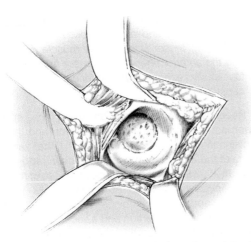

Fig. 4. Exposure of the acetabulum for minimally invasive total hip arthroplasty. (*From* Rachbauer F, Krismer M. Minimalinvasive Hüftendoprothetik über den anterioren Zugang. Oper Orthop Traumatol 2008;20:245; with permission.)

from a minimally invasive approach using these surgical routes of access are limited, essentially, to a shorter skin incision. Even though there still is no universally accepted definition for "minimally invasive total hip arthroplasty," the aim remains clear: a focus on minimizing tissue trauma to accelerate rehabilitation, thus giving a definition by purpose. Because it is a muscle-sparing, not a muscle-splitting, approach, the anterior approach has been used consistently for the implantation of a hip prosthesis.

To fulfill the promises of reducing soft tissue trauma, the concept of tissue preservation must be applied to each of the layers around the hip joint, the skin, the muscles, the joint capsule and

the nerves, and vessels within. An optimal approach should deliver a short skin incision; prevent muscle splitting and/or detachment, and provide possible preservation of the joint capsule. The anterior approach allows these goals to be accomplished.

To approach the acetabulum, posterior incisions require splitting the gluteus maximus muscle and tenotomy of the external rotators and part of quadratus femoris. Lateral approaches split, detach, and crush the gluteus minimus and medius muscles. Splitting of the gluteus maximus muscle may lead to partial denervation, because splitting cuts through portions of the inferior gluteal nerve. Lateral approaches often can lead to lesions of branches of the superior gluteal nerve with possible weakening of the gluteal abductors. Furthermore, in a large number of patients, the reattached abductor muscles do not heal onto the greater trochanter. Ruptures of insufficiently reattached muscle are a known medium-term complication of transgluteal approaches.[47]

For access to the femoral canal, the greater trochanter must be osteotomized or the femur must be rotated internally or externally. Anterior and lateral approaches allow the preservation of the external rotators as they follow their natural course. The necessary further step is levering the entrance of the femur to the level of the skin. Double-incision approaches try to obviate levering by entering the femoral canal through the gluteal muscles, accepting as a necessary consequence any collateral damage to the split gluteal muscles and risking possible detachment of the piriformis muscle.[48] Visual accessibility of the femur is compromised also. The extent of leverage might be reduced by splitting or

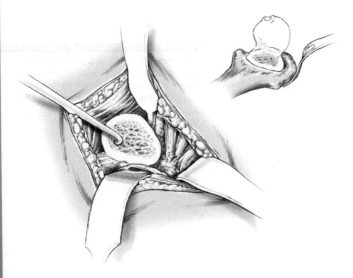

Fig. 5. Exposure of the femur for minimally invasive total hip arthroplasty. (*From* Rachbauer F, Krismer M. Minimalinvasive Hüftendoprothetik über den anterioren Zugang. Oper Orthop Traumatol 2008;20:246; with permission.)

detaching the tensor fasciae latae muscle. To lever the femur, posterior approaches mandate detachment of external rotators and proximal adductors. Lateral approaches require tenotomy of the external rotators, whereas anterior approaches allow their preservation.

The use of an orthopedic traction table has been advocated to facilitate delivery of the femur through an anterior approach. Orthopedic tables in trauma units serve to reduce dislocations of fracture ends by traction. As in lateral and posterior approaches, levering the femur for implantation of the femoral component does not mandate traction. Therefore, the orthopedic table serves as an operative assistant to hold the leg and is dispensable.

Additionally, the orthopedic table may not overcome insufficient release of the proximal femur despite its elongated lever arm, as evidenced by reports of ankle fractures and knee sprains.[39,40,49] The key to successful delivery lies in exact anatomic knowledge of the insertion and direction of action of the external rotators, including their relation to the joint capsule and the gluteal muscles. A stepwise release starting with capsulotomy (not capsulectomy) and, when necessary, proceeding with the release of the conjoint tendon of the obturator internus and gemelli tendons allows sufficient exposure of the proximal femur. Very rarely is the release of the piriformis tendon needed.

Anterior approaches are prone to lesions of the lateral cutaneous femoral nerve. To lower that risk, an incision site located more laterally on the belly of the tensor fasciae latae muscle has been advocated.

The anterior approach is a safe, reliable, and feasible technique for total hip arthroplasty, permitting optimal soft tissue preservation. Since Hueter first described this interval, many surgeons have approached the hip anteriorly to perform a myriad of surgical procedures. The anterior approach allows optimal muscle preservation, and it is the only truly internervous approach to the hip. An appreciation for the evolution of the anterior approach to the hip will help the orthopedic community understand these advantages and why so many have used this approach in the treatment of hip pathology and for the implantation total hip arthroplasty.

REFERENCES

1. Calandruccio R. Voies d'abord de la hanche. Milano, Barcelona, Bonn. In: Roy-Camille R, Laurin CA, Riley LH, editors, Membre inférieur, Atlas de Chirugie orthopédique, vol. 3. Paris: Masson; 1991. p. 65–70.

2. Wikipedia. Available at: http://de.wikipedia.org/wiki/Carl_Hueter. Accessed May 31, 2008.

3. König F. Nekrolog. Langenbecks Arch Surg 1882; 17(3–4):421–30.

4. Hueter C. Fünfte abtheilung: die verletzung und krankheiten des hüftgelenkes, neunundzwanzigstes capitel. In: Hueter C, editor. Grundriss der chirurgie. 2nd edition. Leipzig: FCW Vogel; 1883. p. 129–200.

5. Vulpius O, Stoffel A. Operationen am hüftgelenk, 2. Orthopädische resektionen und mobilisierung des hüftgelenkes, 2. Vorderer hautschnitt nach hueter. In: Vulpius O, Stoffel A, editors. Orthopädische Operationslehre. 3rd edition. Stuttgart: Ferdinand Enke; 1924. p. 435–6.

6. W.A.L. In memoriam Dr. MN Smith-Petersen. J Bone Joint Surg Br 1953;35:482–4.

7. Smith-Petersen MN. A new supra-articular subperiosteal approach to the hip joint. J Bone Joint Surg Am 1917;s2–15:592–5.

8. Lance M. Constitution dúne buteé ostéoplastique dans les luxations et sub-luxations congénitales de la hanche. Presse Méd 1925;33:922–31.

9. Chiron P, Arthroscopy, shelf and core decompression: minimal access conservative hip surgery. Maîtrise orthopédique April 2003. Available at: http://www.maitrise-orthop.com/viewPage_us.do?id=945. Accessed September 11, 2008.

10. Salter RB. Innominate osteotomiy in the treatment of congenital dislocation and subluxation of the hip. J Bone Joint Surg Br 1961;43:518–39.

11. Pemberton PA. Pericapsular osteotomy of the ilium for treatment of congenital subluxation and dislocation of the hip. J Bone Joint Surg Am 1965;47: 65–86.

12. Ganz R, Klaue K, Vinh TS, et al. A new periacetabular osteotomy for the treatment of hip dysplasias. Technique and preliminary results. Clin Orthop Relat Res 1988;232:26–36.

13. Cubbins WR, Callahan JJ, Scuderi CS. Fractures of the neck of the femur. Surg Gynecol Obstet 1939; 68;87.

14. Fahey JJ. Surgical approaches to bone and joints. Surg Clin North Am 1949;29:65.

15. Levine MA. A treatment of central fractures of the acetabulum: a case report. J Bone Joint Surg Am 1943;25:902–6.

16. Judet R, Judet J, Letournel E. Fractures of the acetabulum: classification and surgical approaches for open reduction: preliminary report. J Bone Joint Surg Am 1964;46:1615–75.

17. Letournel E. Acetabulum fractures: classification and management. Clin Orthop Relat Res 1980;151: 81–106.

18. Griffin DB. Beaulé PE, Matta JM. Safety and efficacy of the extended iliofemoral approach in the

treatment of complex fractures of the acetabulum. J Bone Joint Surg Br 2005;87–B:1391–6.

19. Enneking WF, Dunham WK. Resection and reconstruction for primary neoplasms involving the innominate bone. J Bone Joint Surg Am 1978;60:731–46.

20. Beaulé PE, Griffin DB, Matta JJ. The Levine anterior approach for total hip replacement as the treatment for an acute acetabular fracture. J Orthop Trauma 2004;18(9):623–9.

21. Smith-Petersen MN. Treatment of malum coxae senilis, old slipped upper femoral epiphysis, intrapelvic protrusion of the acetabulum, and coxa plana by means of acetabuloplasty. J Bone Joint Surg Am 1936;18:869–80.

22. Ganz R, Gill TJ, Gautier E, et al. Surgical dislocation of the adult hip. J Bone Joint Surg Br 2001;83B(8): 1119–24.

23. Philippon MJ, Stubbs AJ, Schenker ML, et al. Arthroscopic management of femoroacetabular impingement: osteoplasty technique and literature review. Am J Sports Med 2007;35(9):1571–80.

24. Clohisy JC, McClure JT. Treatment of anterior femoroacetabular impingement with combined hip arthroscopy and limited anterior decompression. Iowa Orthop J 2005;25:164–71.

25. Hisashi I, Torii S, Hasegawa Y, et al. Indications and results of vascularized pedicle iliac bone graft in avascular necrosis of the femoral head. Clin Orthop Relat Res 1993;295:281–8.

26. Kirkaldy-Willis WH. Ischio-femoral arthrodesis of the hip in tuberculosis. An anterior approach. J Bone Joint Surg 1950;32–B:187–92.

27. Matta JM, Siebenrock KA, Gautier E, et al. Hip fusion through an anterior approach with the use of a ventral plate. Clin Orthop Relat Res 1997;337: 129–39.

28. Smith-Peterson MN. Approach to and exposure of the hip joint for mold arthroplasty. J Bone Joint Surg Am 1949;31:40–6.

29. Judet J, Judet R. The use of an artificial femoral head for arthroplasty of the hip joint. J Bone Joint Surg Br 1950;32-B:166–73.

30. O'Brien RM. The technic for insertion of femoral head prosthesis by the straight anterior or hueter approach. Clin Orthop 1955;6:22–6.

31. Luck JV. An approach for hip construction. Broad visualization without osteotomy of the greater trochanter. Clin Orthop Relat Res 1973;91:70–85.

32. Charnley J. Low friction arthroplasty of the hip. Theory & Practice. London: Springer; 1979.

33. Wagner H. Surface replacement arthroplasty of the hip. Clin Orthop Relat Res 1978;134:102–30.

34. Judet J, Judet H. Voie d'abord antérieure dans l'arthroplastie totale de la hanche. Presse Méd 1985; 14:1031–3.

35. Light TR, Keggi KJ. Anterior approach to hip arthroplasty. Clin Orthop Relat Res 1980;152:255–60.

36. Kennon RE, Keggi JM, Wetmore RS, et al. Total hip arthroplasty through a minimally invasive anterior surgical approach. J Bone Joint Surg Am 2003; 85-A(Suppl 4):39–48.

37. Berger RA. Total hip arthroplasty using the minimally invasive two-incision approach. Clin Orthop Relat Res 2003;417:232–41.

38. Küntscher G. Intramedullary surgical technique and its place in orthopaedic surgery: my present concept. J Bone Joint Surg Am 1965;47:809–18.

39. Siguier T, Siguier M, Brumpt B. Mini-incision anterior approach does not increase dislocation rate: a study of 1037 total hip replacements. Clin Orthop Relat Res 2004;426:164–73.

40. Matta JM, Shahrdar C, Ferguson T. Single-incision anterior approach for total hip arthroplasty on an orthopaedic table. Clin Orthop Relat Res 2005; 441:115–24.

41. Rachbauer F, Nogler M, Mayr E, et al. Minimally invasive single incision anterior approach for total hip arthroplasty—early results. In: Hozack WJ, Krismer M, Nogler M, et al, editors. Minimally invasive total joint arthroplasty. Berlin: Springer; 2004. p. 54–9.

42. Rachbauer F, Nogler M, Krismer M, et al. Minimal invasive total hip arthroplasty via direct anterior single approach [Paper No 141]. In: Proceedings of the 2005 annual meeting of the American Academy of Orthopaedic Surgeons. Washington, DC: American Academy of Orthopaedic Surgeons; 2005. p. 355.

43. Rachbauer F. Minimal invasive Hüftendoprothetik über einen direkten vorderen Zugang. Orthopäde 2005;34:1103–10 [in German].

44. Rachbauer F. Minimal-invasive Hüftendoprothetik. Der vordere Zugang. Orthopäde 2006;35:723–30 [in Germen].

45. Rachbauer F, Rosiek R, Nogler M, et al. The benefits of the direct anterior approach in minimally invasive THA [Paper No 202]. In: Proceedings of the 2006 annual meeting of the American Academy of Orthopaedic Surgeons. Chicago: American Academy of Orthopaedic Surgeons; 2006. p. 480.

46. Rachbauer F, Krismer M. Minimalinvasive Hüftendoprothetik über den anterioren Zugang. Oper Orthop Traumatol 2008;20:239–51.

47. Stähelin T, Drittenbass L, Hersche D, et al. Failure of capsular enhanced short external rotator repair after total hip replacement. Clin Orthop Relat Res 2004; 420:199–204.

48. Pagnago MW. Minimally invasive THA: two incision approach in 2007. In: Programs and Abstracts of the Thirteenth Combined Open Meeting Hip Society and the American Association of Hip and Knee Surgeons. San Diego (CA), February 18, 2007.

49. Sariali E, Leonard P, Mamoudy P. Dislocation after total hip arthroplasty using Hueter anterior approach. J Arthroplasty 2008;23:266–72.

Direct Anterior Approach for Total Hip Arthroplasty

Benjamin Bender, MD[a,*], Michael Nogler, MD, MA, MAS, MSc[b],
William J. Hozack, MD[a,*]

KEYWORDS

- Single incision
- Interval between tensor fasciae latae/gluteus medius and rectus femoris/sartorius
- Lateral femoral cutaneous nerve (LFCN)
- Specialized instruments
- Sparing of the abductor muscles

Total hip arthroplasty (THA) is considered one of the most successful surgical procedures, because it relieves pain, restores mobility, and improves quality of life for patients who had previously incapacitating arthritis. In the United States almost 250,000 total hip replacements are performed annually, and this number is expected to rise to 572,000 (plus another 97,000 revisions) by 2030. There are numerous causes of hip arthritis, including childhood disorders (such as development dysplasia of the hip, Perthes disease, and slipped capital femoral epiphysis), inflammatory arthritis, osteonecrosis, trauma, and infection. For most patients, however, a growing body of evidence suggests that subtle morphologic changes in the hip, such as acetabular retroversion, mild acetabular dysplasia, and subtle forms of epiphyseal slippage are the underlying causes of hip arthritis.[1–7]

The success of operative treatment depends on a quick recovery of limb function and the safety and reproducibility of the procedure as well as on the alleviation of associated pain.[2,5,8,9] The concept of minimally invasive surgery was introduced to orthopedics in the 1970s by Watanabe[10] in association with arthroscopy. Minimally invasive surgery is defined as a surgical technique performed through a short skin incision to minimize injury to muscles and/or bones. The term "minimally invasive" does not necessarily indicate a short scar but rather refers to minimal damage to soft tissues, particularly muscles and their insertions.[1,7,11,12] Every injury to a muscle or its attachment is associated with decreased muscle strength and impaired proprioception.

Muscle protection translates into accelerated rehabilitation, which in turn potentially enables the patient to be discharged from the surgical ward and to start rehabilitation faster. In a standard surgical approach the size of the incision is dictated by the requirements during the surgery; with minimally invasive techniques the size of the surgical approach has much more fixed parameters.[1,7,8,13–16] Minimally invasive approaches include the posterior, anterolateral, direct anterior, and two-incision approaches. During recent years the orthopedic community has witnessed an immense interest in minimally invasive surgery, particularly for THA, Although the long-term outcomes of minimally invasive THA are unknown at this point, some studies have reported short-term benefits, stating that minimally invasive THA reduces intraoperative blood loss, reduces perioperative pain, results in faster recovery, shortens

[a] Department of Orthopaedic Surgery, Rothman Institute of Orthopaedics, Thomas Jefferson University Hospital, 925 Chestnut Street, Philadelphia, PA 19107, USA
[b] Department of Orthopaedic Surgery, Medical University of Innsbruck, Anichstrasse 35, A-6020-Innsbruck, Austria
* Corresponding authors.
E-mail addresses: BenjaminBender@hotmail.com (B. Bender); william.hozack@rothmaninstitute.com (W.J. Hozack).

Orthop Clin N Am 40 (2009) 321–328
doi:10.1016/j.ocl.2009.01.003

hospital stay, and provides better incision cosmetics.[1,2,6,8,16–19] Other studies, however, refute the benefits of minimally invasive THA, reporting higher complication rates, and a worse cosmetic appearance for the incision.[3,9,20] In addition, the learning curve connected with minimally invasive surgery is steep, and mastering the skill frequently is an on-going process. Also, it is possible that confounding factors such as patient selection, patient and family education, accelerated rehabilitation, and better pain control may play important roles in influencing the outcome of minimally invasive THA.[1,4,5,13,18,21,22]

The anterior approach best follows the principles of minimally invasive surgery, because it makes possible the implantation of a hip prosthesis with minimal damage to muscles or their insertions. This approach was described first by Robert Judet in 1947 as a modification of the Smith-Peterson approach. Judet used an orthopedic table with indirect traction applied to both feet, because traction applied to the lower limbs combined with traction and simultaneous external rotation and hyperextension in the hip joint of the treated limb facilitates hip joint dislocation. Current modifications of the technique do not require an orthopedic table and traction to the lower limbs.

The procedure now can be performed on a flattop table. Hyperextension is obtained before the femoral preparation and is achieved by manipulating the table to break at the level of the pelvis and hyperextend the legs. The direct anterior approach is an internervous plane surgical approach. Access to the joint capsule is achieved through the septum between the tensor fasciae latae (TLF) and gluteus medius (innervated by the superior gluteal nerve) and the rectus femoris of the quadriceps femoris muscle and the sartorius (innervated by the femoral nerve).[12,13,18,23,24]

The use of appropriate instruments significantly facilitates prosthesis implantation and, more importantly, reduces the risk of complication. The procedure also is facilitated by the use of a fiberoptic light source attached to retractors.[23,25]

INDICATIONS/CONTRAINDICATIONS

Indications for using the minimally invasive technique comprise moderate degenerative changes in the hip joint of various etiologies requiring total hip replacement. The ideal patient is a flexible, non-muscular patient with a valgus femoral neck and good femoral offset. Not every surgeon can perform the minimally invasive procedure, because it requires excellent manual skills and knowledge of anatomy, as well as experience in performing conventional hip joint surgery so

that the operator can widen the approach appropriately if need be. An efficient and experienced operating team, including the assistants and adjunct personnel, also is of great importance.

Initially the surgeon should use the approach only for slender patients who have a body mass index under 30 (less than degree I obesity) with moderately developed subcutaneous tissue and muscles around the joint. As the surgeon develops experience, this approach can be used for virtually all patients.

About 80% of the authors' primary total hip replacements are done through the direct anterior approach, but alternative approaches should be considered if there is a significant femoral bone deformity. Ideal candidates for the surgery are patients who have moderately developed subcutaneous tissue and muscles and no femoral deformities. Local skin irritation or infection at the site of the surgical is considered an absolute contraindication. An obese patient who has soft tissue folds that overhang the incision area is at a higher risk of wound-healing complications. The exposure is more difficult in muscular patients (as probably is true for all approaches to the hip), but the approach is not absolutely contraindicated in these patients.

The lack of appropriate instrumentation is also considered a contraindication. The direct anterior approach requires the availability of specially curved, angled, or offset instruments.[5,6,12,17,18,21,22,25–27]

The direct anterior approach can be used for revision surgery as well, but distal exposure of the femur requires that the incision be curved laterally to prevent injury to the femoral nerve and vessels. A partial release of the TFL muscle's origin gives straight access to the femur. Lateral access to the femur can be achieved by a dorsolateral extension of the incision or by a second lateral incision dorsal to the lateral vastus muscle. In revision THA the direct anterior approach is particularly useful for isolated simple acetabular revisions.[3,17,18,23]

POSITIONING AND DRAPING

A standard operating table is used. The table can be broken at the level of the hip joint to hyperextend both legs. The patient is positioned in the supine position, and the operative leg is draped. The supine position achieves a stable pelvis and allows easy measurement of leg length. The opposite leg is supported by an additional arm board that is attached to the table, making hyperabduction of the opposite leg during femoral exposure easier. The authors drape only the operated leg, but some surgeons drape both legs; doing so allows the operated leg to be crossed under the opposite leg during the surgical exposure of the femur.

SKIN INCISION

The position of the skin incision is determined by palpating the anterior superior iliac spine (ASIS) from below. From this point, measure 3 cm laterally and 3 cm distally to find the starting point and orientate the incision along the longitudinal axis of the TFL muscle. Keep the initial incision small (8–10 cm), but do not hesitate to extend it as needed (**Fig. 1**). Lengthen the incision distally to increase acetabular exposure and proximally to increase exposure of the femur. The site of the incision is located much more laterally than the site of the incision in the original Smith-Petersen approach. Another method for finding the incision site is to draw a line between the ASIS and the greater tuberosity. The proximal extent of the incision starts on this line about halfway between the two landmarks. The incision should angled gradually toward the greater tuberosity rather than going straight distally. In the area of the incision, vessels perforating the iliotibial band can be found and must be cauterized.

INTERMUSCULAR PORTAL

The lateral femoral circumflex nerve and its branches lie along the surface of the sartorius muscle. As an additional step to protect the lateral femoral circumflex nerve, the authors recommend incising the TFL sharply at its midpoint for the length of the muscle and performing a strictly subfascial exposure. Elevation of the medial aspect of the superficial TFL fascia reveals a fat layer medially. This fat layer defines the Smith Peterson interval.

Inserting an index finger posteriorly at this point allows the surgeon to reach the superior aspect of the hip joint capsule. An alternative technique is to identify the fascia of the gluteus medius muscle; it has a consistently whiter, more fascial appearance. Immediately medial is the tensor fascia (**Fig. 2**). At this point, a curved retractor is placed medial to the TFL and gluteus minimus, near the superior hip joint capsule. Using a finger, carefully separate the remaining fibers of the sartorius and TFL to expose the Smith Peterson interval fully. Place a second sharp retractor at the distal part of the incision near the greater trochanter. Using a wide rake or Hibbs retractor, pull the sartorius and rectus medially. Using this instrumentation and placement of the retractors, exposes the lateral aspect of the hip joint through the direct anterior interval; the TFL is located laterally to the exposure, and the rectus and sartorius are located medially. The ascending branches of the lateral circumflex vessels must be identified and cauterized, sutured, or clipped. These branches vary in number. This interval is truly intermuscular and internerval; all the medial muscles are supplied by the femoral nerve, and all the lateral muscles are supplied by the superior gluteal nerve. Once the lateral circumflex vessels are cauterized, the surgeon can incise the fascial layer between the rectus and the TFL to reveal the lateral vastus muscle. The fascia between rectus and capsule is dissected with the electro-coagulation until the precapsular fat pad is visible. The hip is flexed

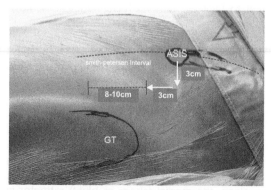

Fig. 1. The site of incision is localized 3 cm lateral and 3 cm distal to the ASIS. Incision length is about 8 to 10 cm. The incision is localized more laterally than the original Smith-Petersen interval to protect the LFCN. (*Courtesy of* M. Nogler, MSc, Innsbruck, Austria.)

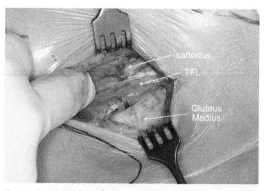

Fig. 2. Precise identification of the TFL is crucial. The index finger is used in a proximal-to-distal movement to palpate the interval between the TFL and sartorius. An alternative way to identify the TFL is by its location medial to the gluteus. The fascia of gluteus medius muscle is whiter than surrounding tissue. (*Courtesy of* M. Nogler, MSc, Innsbruck, Austria.)

during this step. A "soft-spot" that offers very little resistance can be palpated just proximal to the lateral vastus muscle. Blunt dissection with a finger or a Cobb instrument can identify the proper location for the retractor. Place another retractor medial to the neck, thus retracting the rectus and sartorius. Either a sharp or blunt retractor can be used.

The distal lateral retractor (in the area of the greater tuberosity) can be removed at this step. After the strong fascia under the rectus is released, the Cobb instrument is used to prepare the space around the ventral rim of the acetabulum. The hip is flexed during this step. A fourth sharp retractor is placed around the ventral rim. A light attachment on this retractor can enhance the visibility of the acetabulum dramatically. If necessary, the rectus fascia can be released further. Afterwards, return the lateral distal retractor to its primary position. If the retractor is placed perpendicularly to the ilioinguinal band and kept under the iliopsoas muscle, injuries of the femoral nerve or the vascular bundle can be avoided (**Fig. 3**).

ANTERIOR CAPSULECTOMY

Start the capsulectomy with a cut laterally along the axis of the femoral neck. Distally, be sure to remove the entire capsule, but do not cut into the lateral vastus, which will cause bleeding. Try to

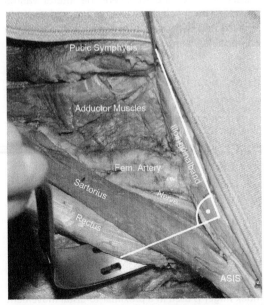

Fig. 3. To avoid injuries to the femoral nerve and vascular bundle, the retractor is placed perpendicular to the ilioinguinal band and is kept under the iliopsoas muscle. (*Courtesy of* M. Nogler, MSc, Innsbruck, Austria.)

cut as far proximally as possible. This ventral capsular flap can be kept in place or removed completely. The inferior or medial retractor then is placed inside the capsule around the femoral neck. In rare cases, if necessary, the reflected head of the rectus can be incised at its capsular insertion. It also is possible to perform a capsulotomy and leave the two flaps created in place.

DOUBLE OSTEOTOMY

Remove the superolateral retractor and place a blunt retractor intracapsularily to protect the tip of the greater trochanter during the osteotomy. Typically, a double osteotomy is performed without dislocating the hip joint. Use the "saddle" between the greater trochanter and the neck as a starting point for the second osteotomy. Perform the definitive osteotomy with a microsaw or a standard power tool using a long, small saw blade. The proximal osteotomy should be done as proximally as possible. The use of longer saw blades increases the risk of cuts into the acetabulum or the tip of the greater trochanter. Perform the second osteotomy 1 cm proximal to the first osteotomy. Make sure the osteotomies are parallel; if a wedge is created, removal of the neck might be difficult. The order of the osteotomies can be reversed based on surgeon preference. When removing the disk and femoral head, be careful not to damage the surrounding musculature on the sharp edges of the cut surfaces. Use the Cobb instrument or a chisel to mobilize the neck disk. Remove the neck disk with a clamp or tenaculum. Gentle traction on the leg will facilitate this step. A corkscrew is used to remove the remaining head. A gentle but constant longitudinal pull is the best technique for removing the head. Anterior acetabular osteophytes may need to be removed first to facilitate femoral head removal. Remove acetabular osteophytes before dislocation. In some cases it is necessary to cut the head ligament before a dislocation is possible. These steps can be made easier by pulling the leg downwards.

ACETABULUM EXPOSURE

For the acetabular preparation, additional light is helpful and can be achieved using a head-mounted light or by placing a localized light source in the wound. While the anterior retractor remains in place, the medial (sharp or blunt) retractor is placed in the area of the transverse ligament medial and inferior to the acetabulum. Incising the medial or inferior capsule facilitates placement of this retractor. Another sharp retractor is placed inside the capsule in the area of the posterolateral acetabulum.

REAMING OF THE ACETABULUM

Standard reamers can be used, but it is extremely helpful to have an offset reamer handle available. The offset reamer handle allows reaming in the correct orientation. Ream the acetabulum to the correct size using the offset reamer.

CUP IMPLANTATION

After the trial, use the curved cup impactor to place the cup. The use of a curved cup impactor is essential for achieving the correct cup orientation (**Fig. 4**). If screws are placed, or a locking screw is inserted, use a flexible screw driver.

LEG POSITIONING AND PROXIMAL FEMORAL EXPOSURE

Place the operated leg in hyperextension, adduction, and externally rotation. The table is broken by about 30° to 40° to accomplish hyperextension. The opposite leg is abducted and placed on the arm board. Alternatively, the opposite leg can be crossed over the operated leg and the assistant's hand to support external rotation. Leave the anterior retractor in place, and remove all other retractors. Grasp the lateral capsular flap with a clamp, and place the femoral elevator behind this flap. Another retractor can be placed against the greater trochanter. This retractor is a custom double-pronged retractor (femoral elevator) that is placed behind the greater trochanter but in front of the gluteus medius muscle. The superolateral capsule is seen as a triangle between the acetabulum and femoral neck.

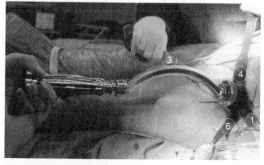

Fig. 4. The curved impactor is used to insert the cup. (1, 3, 4) A sharp Narrow Hohman retractor. (6) Double-pronged Femoral Elevator. (*Courtesy of M. Nogler, MSc, Innsbruck, Austria.*)

This flap must be detached carefully from the neck and should be removed completely. If cuts are made in the posterior capsular fat pad, there is no risk of injuring the short external rotators. Place a bone hook inside the femoral cavity in the calcar area of the femoral neck and lift upward and laterally simultaneously to ensure the greater trochanter is not behind the acetabulum. Place the femoral elevator dorsally to the greater trochanter and be sure to push all attached muscles posteriorly. Use a placed proximally to the lesser trochanter retractor in the calcar area to retract the medial soft tissue. Remove all remnants of the dorsal lateral capsule at the femoral neck.

Additional release of the posterior structure may be required to achieve proper femoral exposure. At the tip of the greater trochanter and in the trochanteric fossa, the attachments of the gluteus minimus, piriformis, gemellus superior, internal obturator, and gemellus inferior can be found. A sharp retractor is placed in the calcar area proximal to the iliopsoas tendon.

Another sharp retractor can be placed laterally at the proximal femur to pull back the lateral soft tissue. After the femur is exposed, the previously mentioned tendons can be released if necessary. Extensive releases are seldom performed; the posterior capsule is never violated, but the piriformis tendon is incised in about 75% of cases.

BROACHING OF THE FEMORAL CANAL

An angled curette is used to open and probe the direction of the femoral canal carefully. A rongeur can be used to extend the opening in the direction of the greater trochanter. Always use the smallest broach available, and always use a double-offset broach handle to broach the femoral canal. Using minimal force, insert the broach handle by hand into the open canal. When the broach is completely aligned with the femur, tap it with the hammer. The double-offset design of the broach handle eases the introduction of the broach because it reduces the need to elevate the proximal femur. This broach design also greatly facilitates surgery for obese and muscular patients when leverage of the proximal femur to skin level cannot be achieved. There are two versions of this broach handle, for the left and the right leg. This lateral offset reduces the need for adduction and elevation of the operated leg. It allows broaching the canal with the proximal femur remaining a few centimeters below skin level (**Fig. 5**). The first broach can be used gently to lateralize further the subsequent broaches. Trialing is done off the broach.

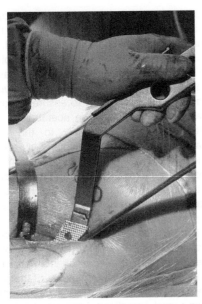

Fig. 5. The double-offset handle is used to facilitate the broaching of the femoral canal. (*Courtesy of* M. Nogler, MSc, Innsbruck, Austria.)

IMPLANTATION, REDUCTION, AND WOUND CLOSURE

The final femoral component should be inserted by hand into the space created by the broaches. A straight impactor cannot be used in the standard fashion. Instead, it should be placed into the femoral stem impaction hole at an angle of 30° to 45°. Angling a standard blunt impactor by 45° directs the forces correctly and completes impaction of the stem. Alternatively, a custom angled impactor can be used. This technique minimizes the risk of medial calcar fracture and ensures lateralization of the femoral component.

The muscular fascia is sutured. Do not place the sutures too far medially; remember, the lateral femoral cutaneous nerve (LFCN) is there. Local anesthetics can be injected regionally, based on the surgeon's preference.

PERIOPERATIVE MANAGEMENT

Sufficient postoperative analgesia is essential. Mobilization is possible within the first 24 hours. When the minimally invasive direct anterior portal approach is used, the reduced muscle damage should result in faster rehabilitation. Whether full weight bearing is allowed is based on the surgeon's preference and the design of the implant being used. The authors' preference is for weight bearing as tolerated.

COMPLICATIONS

In comparison with open approaches in general, the direct anterior approach preserves muscle structures well. Complications involving muscular damage, especially dislocation, should not be expected using this approach, if implants are placed correctly.[24] There is almost no risk of injuring the sciatic nerve, but the femoral nerve is exposed to a higher risk of injury because it lies close to the surgical field. Careful use and placement of the curved retractors avoids damage to this nerve. To protect femoral nerve branches, any preparation of the femur distal to the lesser trochanter should be performed from a lateral approach.

A complication specific to this approach is the damage to the LFCN. The location of this nerve and the number of its branches can vary widely among patients. If a small lateral branch of the LFCN runs across the TFL, it usually is very hard to detect, and it is almost impossible to avoid cutting it accidentally. Such a dissection of the LFCN branch results in numbness around the incision. Damaging the main trunk of the nerve results in numbness in the lateral-distal thigh area. If damage to the main trunk occurs, a very unpleasant complication that can develop is meralgia paraesthetica.[28]

In most cases of injury to LFCN, patients are pain-free immediately postoperatively but develop severe pain in the anterolateral aspect of the thigh a few weeks after the surgery. In most of the revised cases, scar tissue around the nerve trunk can be detected. Damage to the main trunk can be avoided by placing the skin incision as laterally as possible, as described earlier. Further protection to the nerve is gained by ensuring that the medial subcutaneous fat pad remains untouched during the whole procedure.

The motor branch of the superior gluteal nerve to TFL can be injured if the dissection is carried in the TFL and not in the appropriate intermuscular portal.

DISCUSSION

The anterior approach has the advantage of preventing injury to muscles and their attachments to the pelvis and femur, helping restore their normal tension immediately on completion of the surgery. Uninjured muscles and muscle attachments significantly improve the dynamic muscular stabilization of the hip joint. An important advantage of this approach in complicated cases (eg proximal femur fractures) is easy access to proximal femur that can be obtained by extending the incision distally, as in the Smith-Peterson technique. Although revision THA in general tends to be more invasive, the direct anterior approach and its extension have the potential to preserve gluteal muscle in revision cases also. If the approach is extended proximally along the iliac crest or distally along the lateral femur, the term "direct anterior" refers to portion of the approach in the area of the hip joint itself, which exploits the interval between the TFL and the rectus femoris. Nevertheless the main advantage of this portal—keeping the gluteal muscles intact—still can be achieved.

The senior author of this article (WJH) conducted a study that enrolled 100 patients who were assigned randomly into two groups. The first group of patients underwent THA through a single-incision modified Smith-Peterson direct anterior approach. The second group received THA through a small-incision anterolateral approach. All patients were treated with exactly the same postoperative rehabilitation and pain management protocols. Evaluation included length of incision, operative time, estimated blood loss, analgesia requirement, need for transfusion, and length of hospital stay. Functional outcome was assessed by the Short Form-36, the Western Ontario and MacMaster Osteoarthritis Index, lower extremity score, linear analog scale assessment, functional independence measure, and Harris Hip Scores. There was a significant improvement in function for all patients in the cohort. Incision length was the same in both groups. The direct anterior group demonstrated significantly better improvement in the SF-36 scores for role limitation ($P = .001$), bodily pain ($P = .001$), and general mental health ($P = .001$) compared with patients in the anterolateral approach group. All other variables showed no statistical difference. Minimally invasive THA performed through a single direct anterior approach seemed to be a viable approach for some patients, showing short-term benefits when compared with the small-incision anterolateral approach.

SUMMARY

Minimally invasive single-incision direct anterior approach surgery is completed through an 8- to 10-cm incision positioned 3 cm distal and lateral to the ASIS. The skin incision is placed more laterally in this approach to protect the branches of the LFCN. Access to the joint capsule is achieved through the interval between the TFL and gluteus medius; the rectus femoris of the quadriceps femoris muscle and the sartorius fat layer defines the Smith Peterson interval. If the retractor is placed

perpendicularly to the ilioinguinal band and kept under the iliopsoas muscle, injuries to the femoral nerve or the vascular bundle can be avoided. The approach requires the use of specialized instruments for proper visualization and implantation of the hip joint. The use of four specially curved retractors reduces pressure on soft tissue and optimizes the surgical area. The ascending branches of the lateral circumflex vessels must be ligated or cauterized. An offset reamer handle and cup impactor are necessary for correct acetabular preparation and implant placement. The anterior approach does not require any detachment of muscle insertions or muscle dissection. The direct anterior approach spares the abductor muscles and hence minimizes the risk of gluteal insufficiency. The table can be broken at the level of the hip joint to hyperextend both legs. An additional arm board supports the abducted leg.

This article describes the surgical technique of the single-incision direct anterior approach. The authors believe the direct anterior approach has significant advantages, including minimal soft tissue trauma, resulting in faster postoperative mobilization and rehabilitation. The small incision scar also results in better cosmesis.

REFERENCES

1. Berger RA, Jacobs JJ, Meneghini RM, et al. Rapid rehabilitation and recovery with minimally invasive total hip arthroplasty. Clin Orthop Relat Res 2004; 429:239–47.
2. Chimento GF, Pavone V, Sharrock N, et al. Minimally invasive total hip arthroplasty: a prospective randomized study. J Arthroplasty 2005;20(2): 139–44.
3. de BJ, Petruccelli D, Zalzal P, et al. Single-incision, minimally invasive total hip arthroplasty: length doesn't matter. J Arthroplasty 2004;19(8):945–50.
4. Parvizi J, Sharkoy PF, Pour AE, et al. Hip arthroplasty with minimally invasive surgery: a survey comparing the opinion of highly qualified experts vs patients. J Arthroplasty 2006;21(6 Suppl 2):38–46.
5. Pour AE, Parvizi J, Sharkey PF, et al. Minimally invasive hip arthroplasty: what role does patient preconditioning play? J Bone Joint Surg Am 2007;89(9): 1920–7.
6. Sculco TP, Jordan LC, Walter WL. Minimally invasive total hip arthroplasty: the Hospital for Special Surgery experience. Orthop Clin North Am 2004; 35(2):137–42.
7. Waldman BJ. Advancements in minimally invasive total hip arthroplasty. Orthopedics 2003; 26(8 Suppl):s833–6.

8. Mow CS, Woolson ST, Ngarmukos SG, et al. Comparison of scars from total hip replacements done with a standard or a mini-incision. Clin Orthop Relat Res 2005;441:80–5.

9. Ogonda L, Wilson R, Archbold P, et al. A minimal-incision technique in total hip arthroplasty does not improve early postoperative outcomes. A prospective, randomized, controlled trial. J Bone Joint Surg Am 2005;87(4):701–10.

10. Watanabe M. Arthroscopy: the present state. Orthop Clin North Am 1979;10(3):505–22.

11. Sculco TP. Minimally invasive total hip arthroplasty: in the affirmative. J Arthroplasty 2004;19(4 Suppl 1): 78–80.

12. Wojciechowski P, Kusz D, Kopec K, et al. Minimally invasive approaches in total hip arthroplasty. Ortop Traumatol Rehabil 2007;9(1):1–7.

13. Sculco TP, Jordan LC. The mini-incision approach to total hip arthroplasty. Instr Course Lect 2004;53: 141–7.

14. Wenz JF, Gurkan I, Jibodh SR. Mini-incision total hip arthroplasty: a comparative assessment of perioperative outcomes. Orthopedics 2002;25(10):1031–43.

15. Wohlrab D, Hagel A, Hein W. [Advantages of minimal invasive total hip replacement in the early phase of rehabilitation]. Z Orthop Ihre Grenzgeb 2004;142(6):685–90 [in German].

16. Wright JM, Crockett HC, Delgado S, et al. Mini-incision for total hip arthroplasty: a prospective, controlled investigation with 5-year follow-up evaluation. J Arthroplasty 2004;19(5):538–45.

17. Kennon R, Keggi J, Zatorski LE, et al. Anterior approach for total hip arthroplasty: beyond the minimally invasive technique. J Bone Joint Surg Am 2004;86-A(Suppl):291–7.

18. Kennon RE, Keggi JM, Wetmore RS, et al. Total hip arthroplasty through a minimally invasive anterior surgical approach. J Bone Joint Surg Am 2003; 85-A(Suppl):439–48.

19. Woolson ST, Mow CS, Syquia JF, et al. Comparison of primary total hip replacements performed with a standard incision or a mini-incision. J Bone Joint Surg Am 2004;86-A(7):1353–8.

20. Hungerford DS. Minimally invasive total hip arthroplasty: in opposition. J Arthroplasty 2004;19(4 Suppl 1):81–2.

21. Klein GR, Parvizi J, Sharkey PF, et al. Minimally invasive total hip arthroplasty: internet claims made by members of the Hip Society. Clin Orthop Relat Res 2005;441:68–70.

22. Light TR, Keggi KJ. Anterior approach to hip arthroplasty. Clin Orthop Relat Res 1980;152:255–60.

23. Hozack WJ. Direct anterior approach for THA. Presented at the 75th Annual AAOS Meeting, San Francisco, March 5–9, 2008.

24. Siguier T, Siguier M, Brumpt B. Mini-incision anterior approach does not increase dislocation rate: a study of 1037 total hip replacements. Clin Orthop Relat Res 2004;426:164–73.

25. Nogler M, Krismer M, Hozack WJ, et al. A double offset broach handle for preparation of the femoral cavity in minimally invasive direct anterior total hip arthroplasty. J Arthroplasty 2006;21(8): 1206–8.

26. Howell JR, Masri BA, Duncan CP. Minimally invasive versus standard incision anterolateral hip replacement: a comparative study. Orthop Clin North Am 2004;35(2):153–62.

27. Inaba Y, Dorr LD, Wan Z, et al. Operative and patient care techniques for posterior mini-incision total hip arthroplasty. Clin Orthop Relat Res 2005;441: 104–14.

28. Grothaus MC, Holt M, Mekhail AO, et al. Lateral femoral cutaneous nerve: an anatomic study. Clin Orthop Relat Res 2005;437:164–8.

Outcomes Following the Single-Incision Anterior Approach to Total Hip Arthroplasty: A Multicenter Observational Study

The Anterior Total Hip Arthroplasty Collaborative (ATHAC) Investigators

KEYWORDS

- Single incision • Anterior approach
- Total hip arthroplasty • Quality of Life
- Function • Outcomes • Technique

Osteoarthritis, the clinical syndrome of joint pain and dysfunction caused by joint degeneration, affects more people than any other joint disease. This burden has been recognized by the United Nations and World Health Organization by endorsing the Bone and Joint Decade 2000–2010. Osteoarthritis disables approximately 10% of people who are older than 60 years, compromises the quality of life of more than 20 million Americans, and costs the United States economy more than $60 billion per year.[1]

Less invasive approaches have become the focus in arthroplasty, with special approaches and specifically designed instruments to accommodate such approaches. The keywords "minimally invasive surgery" in the medical database PubMed retrieves over 12,000 articles on this topic, of which 11,000 have been published in the past 2 years. An Internet search (Google) reveals over 90,000 hits on "minimally invasive hip surgery," of which 50% have occurred in the past 2 years.

Commonly reported single-incision less-invasive techniques include the anterior approach, the mini-Watson-Jones approach, the trochanteric flake technique, and the miniposterior and mini-posterolateral approaches.[2–9] Dual-incision approaches incorporate two mini-incisions (one anterior-based and one posterior-based).[4,5] This relative explosion of information has further confused the subject matter. Few large series and few small trials exist to provide patients and surgeons sufficient evidence to guide their treatments.

Among these approaches, the direct anterior, intermuscular approach to the hip has several

The study was funded by a research grant from DePuy. The Sponsor was not involved in the design of study, its conduct, the analysis, manuscript writing, or the decision to publish the results. No Sponsor representatives participated in any of the study committees.

* Mohit Bhandari, MD, MSc, member of ATHAC, McMaster University, 293 Wellington Street North, Suite 110, Hamilton, ON, L8L 2X2, Canada.
E-mail address: bhandam@mcmaster.ca

Orthop Clin N Am 40 (2009) 329–342
doi:10.1016/j.ocl.2009.03.001

potential advantages, including preservation of muscle attachments to bone, improved dynamic hip stability, and decreased risk of hip dislocation after surgery.[10–14] The first hip arthroplasty performed through this approach was by Robert Judet in 1947 at Hospital Raymond Poincare in Garches, outside Paris. A Judet acrylic prosthesis was implanted. Judet referred to the surgical approach as the "Hueter Approach." The anterior intermuscular approach has been the subject of two very large observational cohort studies.[10–13] Siguier and colleagues[10] have reported on a series of 1,037 patients treated with the anterior approach to total hip arthroplasty (THA) with an orthopedic table. Keggi and colleagues[11] have also reported a series of 2,132 primary THAs performed via the anterior approach to THA, but without the specific aid of an orthopedic table.[12] Keggi's study reported a dislocation rate of 1.3% and excellent early patient function. Whether the results of this muscle-sparing approach can be extrapolated to surgeons with less experience remains unknown when compared to posterior-muscle splitting or lateral-abductor splitting approaches.

The Anterior Total Hip Arthroplasty Collaborative (ATHAC) is a multicenter research group with an interest in cooperative research toward improving knowledge about the surgical technique (for a list of ATHAC members, see Appendix 1). The current study was conducted to determine outcomes following elective THA using the anterior surgical approach.

METHODS

The investigators conducted a multicenter cohort study of 1,152 patients across nine clinical sites across the United States, evaluating complications and function associated with the anterior approach to THA. The study was coordinated and data analyzed by an independent methods center outside the United States (**Fig.1**). This study was conducted by ATHAC.

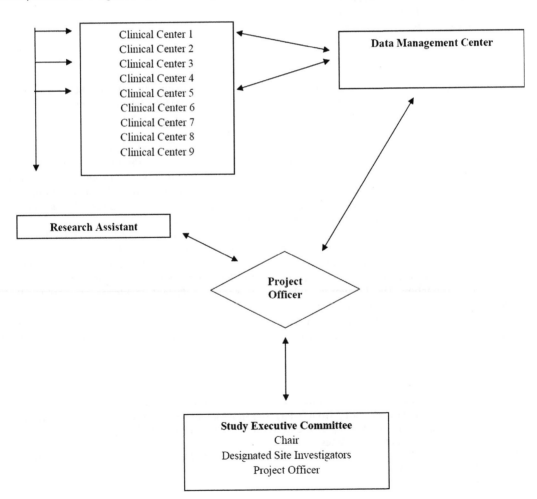

Fig. 1. Study organization.

Eligibility Criteria

Patients were considered to be eligible for the study if they were adults admitted with a primary diagnosis of hip arthritis (ie, diagnosis confirmed radiographically and clinically) and, as a result, were operatively managed with the anterior approach to THA. Patients managed with alternative approaches, revision arthroplasty, and those patients with inadequate records were excluded.

Intervention

Briefly, after administration of general or regional anesthesia, the patient is placed in the supine position on an orthopedic table (eg, Tasserit table, OSI ProFX, or HANA table). The normal incision starts 2-cm to 3-cm posterior and slightly distal to the anterior superior iliac spine. This straight incision extends in a distal and slightly posterior direction to a point 2-cm to 3-cm anterior to the greater trochanter. After incision of the skin and subcutaneous area, the tensor can be seen through the translucent fascia lata. The fascia lata is incised over the tensor and continued distal and proximal to the ends of the skin incision. The sartorius and rectus femorus muscles are retracted medially with a cobra retractor. The lateral femoral circumflex vessels are identified as they cross the distal portion of the wound. These vessels are clamped, cauterized, and transected. The hip capsule is incised and the hip joint is exposed. Details of the full surgical technique are presented in Appendix 2.

Case Report Forms

The investigators collected information about the patients, implants, and procedure. The patient's date of birth, gender, ethnicity, occupation, height, weight, body mass index (BMI), comorbidities (ie, cardiovascular, respiratory, psychiatric, neurologic, genitourinary, gastrointestinal, musculoskeletal, previous lower extremity surgery, and so forth), American Society of Anesthesiologists (ASA) classification, and preoperative diagnosis (ie, osteoarthritis, avascular necrosis, rheumatoid arthritis, septic osteoarthritis, posttrauma, ankylosing spondylitis) were recorded for each patient to provide a depiction of the patient population studied. The following surgical information was abstracted from each patient's medical records: side of hip surgically treated, age at surgery, whether the surgery was a primary THA or if there was a previous surgery on the affected hip, the surgical technique used (ie, length of incision, operative duration, C-arm total time, and other factors), type of anesthesia (ie, general or regional), the estimated blood loss, the acetabular cup position (ie, acetabular inclination/abduction and acetabular anteversion), and the leg-length discrepancy (ie, shorter, longer, or none). Each patient's acetabular and femoral implant information was recorded. Characteristics, such as if bone grafting of the acetabulum was performed, the acetabular implant outer and inner diameter, liner, type (ie, cemented or press-fit), company, and brand were collected, as well as the femoral implant's head and stem size, neck angle, type, and company and brand.

Outcomes

Given the study design, not all study outcome measures were collected at each participating site. Outcomes available at all participating sites included the number of postoperative days in the hospital, the patient's disposition following discharge from the hospital (ie, home, rehabilitation center, aging and long-term care, skilled nursing facility, none), any assistive devices given at discharge and the time it took the patient to discard the assistive devices, revision surgeries, and complications. Outcomes available at few sites included functional outcome indices, such as the Western Ontario McMaster Osteoarthritis index (WOMAC).[15] The investigators varied and reported the denominator for each reported outcome as appropriate.

Data Collection

Data abstraction was conducted using one of two methods. The majority of the centers retained all patient information in personal and medical records. There were a few clinical sites that recorded all information into an electronic database. Each patient's demographic, surgical, and outcome data was recorded using study-specific case-report forms (CRFs).

Seven of the nine participating centers elected to have their own research staff complete the data abstraction. CRFs were shipped to each site and any questions regarding the data abstraction process or completion of CRFs were addressed with regular site contact by the methods center coordinator. Upon receipt, completed patient CRFs were reviewed by the methods center coordinator for missing or inconsistent values. Three centers required site visits by the methods center coordinator to assist with CRF completion.

Pilot Testing and Site Visits

Before the administration of the CRFs to all participating centers, the methods center coordinator conducted a pilot data-abstraction site visit to one of the clinical centers. A random sample of 100 patient records were abstracted; 84 patients were found to be eligible and 16 were excluded. The piloted CRFs were revised to include patients that underwent bilateral THA, data points were rearranged to make data abstraction as painless as possible, and other minor changes were also implemented.

Data Analysis

Sample size calculation

To have sufficient sample size to conduct regression analyses exploring baseline variable association ($n = 10$) with the presence or absence of complications, the investigators required approximately 100 events (ie, 10 events per variable included in the analysis). Given a plausible complication rate of 10%, the investigators required at least 1,000 patients for the study. The sample size was further adjusted to account for ineligible charts (20%). Thus, 1,200 patients was a reasonable sample size to assure sufficient study power (80%) for the regression analysis.

The investigators further planned to compare outcomes among surgeons with 100 or fewer cases with surgeons with greater than 100 cases. If one anticipates a learning curve in complication rates, it remains plausible that a 40% reduction in complication risk could occur over and after the first 100 cases. The investigators assumed a 10% baseline complication risk and thus a reduction from 15% to 9% constituted a 40% reduction in risk. Assuming an alpha = 0.05, and a study power = 0.80, 460 patients were required per arm of the study.

Statistical analysis

The investigators reported baseline patient characteristics as mean and standard deviations (SD) (or median and interquartile range, if the data were skewed) for continuous data, and proportions and percentages for categorical data. Independent sample t-tests were conducted for continuous data and chi-square for categorical data to compare the baseline characteristics (ie, across less and more experienced surgeons). P-values were corrected for multiple testing when multiple tests of association were conducted.

A regression analyses was conducted to evaluate variables associated with patient complications, pain and function, and days in hospital. Univariable analyses were conducted and those variables that revealed association (at the $P<0.1$ level) were entered into a multivariable model. Logistic regression with odds ratios and their associated 95% confidence intervals were reported.

RESULTS
Study Population

Across nine participating sites, 1,152 eligible patients who underwent a total of 1,277 THAs using the anterior approach were identified (**Fig. 2**). Patients were a mean age 65 years, predominantly Caucasian, with a mean BMI of 28. The majority of patients had a preoperative diagnosis of osteoarthritis. One hundred twenty-five patients underwent bilateral hip arthroplasty (**Table 1**). Across centers, patients did not differ by gender or BMI; however, there were differences in mean patient age ($P<0.01$) and ASA class ($P<0.001$) across centers.

Technical Aspects of Surgery

Surgeons operated on patients for an average 95 minutes, with a mean-incision length under 10 cm and 30 seconds of fluoroscopic time (**Table 2**). A variety of implant vendors were used, with almost all surgeons using a press-fit femoral stem (**Table 3**). The bearing surface was most commonly a metal on cross-linked polyethylene (**Table 4**). The most common femoral head sizes used were 28 mm (39.8%) and 32 mm (50.3%). Leg length discrepancy averaged 0.4 cm.

Hospital Stay and Assistive Devices

Patients were in hospital for a mean 3.6 days, with the majority discharged to home (82.6%) (**Table 5**). All but 24 patients used an assistive device at discharge from hospital. The most common devices were walkers and crutches (see **Table 5**). Assistive devices were discontinued at a mean 21 (median, 14) days; however, 80% of patients no longer used an assistive device by 4 days after hospital discharge.

Revision Surgery

Thirty-five patients required a reoperation after the index procedure (**Table 6**). Seventeen of the revisions were the result of aseptic loosening of the prosthesis. Of eight dislocations, three required implant revision (one liner, one femoral head, and one stem); five were treated with closed reduction in the operating room. Leg-length discrepancy required reoperation in three patients.

Regression analysis suggested a strong association between the need for revision surgery and surgeon (center effect) ($P<0.001$).

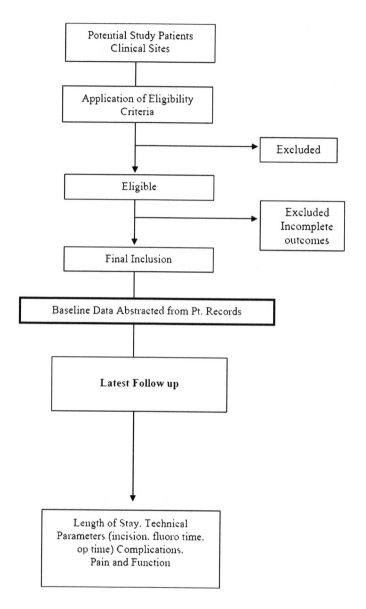

Fig. 2. Study flow.

Complications

Table 7 details both musculoskeletal and general medical complications. Twenty patients experienced cardiovascular complications, 3 psychologic, 8 neurologic, 27 wound-related, 6 genitourinary, and 36 miscellaneous (anemia, nausea, edema, hypokalemia). One patient died in the study cohort of 1,152 patients.

Regression analysis suggested significant associations between the presence of a complication and three variables: length of hospital stay (odds ratio = 1.2, $P<0.001$), BMI (odds ratio = 1.1, $P = 0.05$), and surgeon/center (odds ratio = 1.3, $P = 0.01$).

The investigators further compared surgeons with 100 or greater case experience (total patients included, 842) versus those with less than 100 case experience (total patients included, 435) on complication rates. Surgeons who had performed less than 100 cases were twofold more likely to have complications in their patients (20.2% versus 9.8%, $P = 0.049$).

Patient Function

Functional outcome was assessed in a subset a centers and patients (**Table 8**). WOMAC-determined pain and function scores plateaued by 3 months. Nonsignificant differences in scores were identified at follow-up visits of 3, 6, 12, 24, and 36 months after the index procedure (**Table 9**). Regression analysis suggested a strong

Table 1
Patient demographics (n = 1,152 patients)

Characteristic		(%)
Sex	Male	47.5%
	Female	52.5%
Age at surgery	Mean (SD)	65.26
		(12.196)
Ethnicity	Caucasian	91.2%
	Asian	1.4%
	Hispanic	3.2%
	African-American	3.2%
	Other	0.9%
Occupation	Employed	32.9%
	Unemployed	0.7%
	Disability	1.9%
	Retired	45.8%
	Student	0.1%
	Unknown	18.6%
Height (inches)	Mean (SD)	67 (4)
Weight (pounds)	Mean (SD)	181 (42)
BMI	Mean (SD)	28 (5)
Comorbidities	Cardiovascular	589 (51.1%)
	Respiratory	115 (10.0%)
	Psychiatric	133 (11.5%)
	Neurologic	79 (6.9%)
	Genitourinary	103 (8.9%)
	Gastrointestinal	136 (11.8%)
	Musculoskeletal	401 (34.8%)
	Previous lower-extremity surgery	265 (23.3%)
ASA classification	Class I	7.0%
	Class II	73.4%
	Class III	18.5%
	Class IV	1.1%
	Class V	0%
	Class VI	0%

Table 2
Surgical data (n = 1,152 patients; n = 1,275 hips)

Characteristic		n (%)
Hip operated on	Left	482 (37.8%)
	Right	545 (42.7%)
	Bilateral	125 (9.8%)
Previous surgery on affected hip		87 (6.8%)
Preoperative diagnosis	Osteoarthritis	93.0%
	Avascular necrosis	3.9%
	Rheumatoid arthritis	0.5%
	Post trauma	1.4%
	Other	1.1%

return to function, and (*iii*) a decline in complications in surgeons with greater than 100 case experiences.

Strengths and Limitations

The current study has several strengths. Participating surgeons across nine hospital sites improved the generalizability (external validity) of

Table 3
Surgical technique

Characteristic	
Length of incision (centimeters) Mean (SD)	9.6 (2.2)
Operative duration (minutes) Mean (SD)	95.3 (34.9)
C-arm total time (seconds) Mean (SD)	30.0 (15.4)
Type of Anesthesia	
General	49.0%
Regional	36.0%
Spinal	13.4%
Epidural	1.6%
Estimated blood loss (cc) Mean (SD)	427.4 (293.2)
Acetabular inclination/ abduction (degrees) Mean (SD)	42.1 (6.6)
Acetabular anteversion (degrees) Mean (SD)	19.2 (7.7)
Leg-length discrepancy (±) (millimeters) Mean (SD)	3.9 (3.5)

association between the need for revision surgery and surgeon (center effect) ($P<0.001$).

DISCUSSION
Summary of Principle Findings

In the cohort of 1,152 patients treated with the anterior approach to THA, the investigators found: (*i*) an acceptable complication profile, (*ii*) an early

Table 4
Implants used

Characteristic		*n* (%)
Acetabulum		
Bone grafting		0.6%
Outer diameter (millimeters)	Mean (SD)	54 (4.0)
Acetabular liner	Neutral	85.2%
	20°	9.1%
	Offset	3.8%
	10°	1.4%
	Other	0.5%
Diameter of acetabular linear	26 mm	0.1%
	28 mm	40.7%
	30 mm	0.1%
	32 mm	50.9%
	36 mm	3.8%
	38 mm	3.5%
	40 mm	0.1%
	44 mm	0.2%
	46 mm	0.3%
	48 mm	0.4%
Type	Press-fit	99.8%
	Cemented	0.2%
Implant company and brand used	Zimmer	39.2%
	Smith & Nephew	21.1%
	PLUS	17.7%
	Stryker	8.3%
	DePuy	7.0%
	Encore	3.9%
	Wright-Medical	2.3%
	Biomet	0.5%
Bearing surface		
Type	Metal-on-crosslinked polyethylene	59.9%
	Ceramic-on-crosslinked polyethylene	17.5%
	Ceramic-on-ceramic	12.9%
	Metal-on-metal	4.8%
	Oxinium-on-crosslinked polyethylene	4.5%
	Ceramic-on-metal	0.4%
Implant company and brand used	Zimmer	51.8%
	Smith & Nephew	30.7%
	Stryker	10.9%
	DePuy	4.6%
	Wright-Medical	1.0%
	Biomet	0.6%
	PLUS	0.3%
	Encore	0.1%
Femur		
Femoral head size	26 mm	0.1%
	28 mm	39.8%
	32 mm	50.3%
	36 mm	4.0%
	38 mm	4.6%
	40 mm	0.2%
	44 mm	0.1%
	46 mm	0.3%
	48 mm	0.5%
	50 mm	0.1%
Implant size (millimeters)	Mean (SD)	5.47 (3.355)
Neck Angle (degrees)	Mean (SD)	128.75 (3.395)
Type	Press-fit	94.6%
	Cemented	5.4%
	Zimmer	41.5%
	PLUS	18.0%
	Stryker	13.1%
	DePuy	8.5%
	Smith & Nephew	8.3%
	Encore	3.4%
	Biomet	4.2%
	Wright-Medical	2.7%
	Centrepulse	0.3%

the findings. The sample size of over 1,000 patients provided sufficient precision for data analysis. Careful attention to data management and independent data analysis from the operating surgeons further improved the validity of the findings. Although attempts were made to improve the quality of the reporting by site visits, when necessary, the findings are limited by the retrospective design. Inconsistencies in reporting also limited assessment of functional scores. Moreover, because of insufficient data, the investigators were unable to evaluate function in the early postoperative period (less than 3 months). Thus, the findings about return to function, while interesting for hypothesis-generation, require further confirmation in prospective studies. In addition, it is not known if some surgeons were selecting patients for the anterior approach.

Relevant Literature

Minimally invasive hip surgery has gained popularity, with several reported techniques including single- and double-incision approaches. Commonly reported single-incision techniques include the anterior approach, the mini-Watson-Jones approach, the trochanteric flake technique, miniposterior and mini-posterolateral approach. Dual-incision approaches

Table 5
Outcome data (discharge and assistive device information)

Characteristic		n (%)
Length of hospital stay	Mean (SD)	3.6 (2.4)
Discharge disposition	Home	82.6%
	Aging and long-term care/skilled nursing facility	8.8%
	Rehabilitation facility	8.5%
	Other	0.1%
Assistive device at discharge	Walker	51.8%
	Crutches	28.4%
	Cane	10.9%
	Assistive device indicated, but not specified	5.7%
	None	2.1%
	One crutch	0.8%
	Wheelchair	0.2%
Time to discard assistive device (days)	Mean (SD)	20.8 (13.7)

incorporate two mini-incisions (one anterior-based and one posterior-based).[2–9]

The miniposterior approach has been the focus of several uncontrolled case series;[16–18] however, little evidence exists to support the use of a muscle-splitting miniposterior incision over

Table 6
Outcome data (revision surgeries) (n = 1,277 hips)

Characteristic	n (%)
Primary revision surgery required[a]	35 (2.7%)
Aseptic loosening	17 (1.3%)
Periprosthetic fracture	9 (0.7%)
Hip dislocation[b]	8 (0.6%)
Infection	3 (0.2%)
Leg-length discrepancy	3 (0.2%)
Secondary revision surgery required[a]	0

[a] Patient may require revision surgery for multiple reasons, so these numbers do not add.
[b] Of eight dislocations treated in the operating room, three (0.2%) required implant revision (one liner, one femoral head, and one stem); five were treated with closed reduction in operating room.

a standard posterior incision. Two randomized trials (Level 1 evidence, therapy) suggest no benefit to the miniposterior incision. A randomized trial of 219 patients treated with a standard posterior incision versus a miniposterior incision found no advantage to the smaller incision in hospital stay or short-term outcomes.[2] Another randomized trial of 135 patients reported similar results. There was no evidence that the mini-incision technique resulted in less bleeding or less trauma to the soft tissues of the hip, factors that would have produced a quicker recovery and a shorter hospital stay, than did the standard technique.[3] By virtue of requiring a posterior incision, the two-incision approach[4,5] also suffers the same limitations of a lack of observable benefit over conventional incisions.

Reports of the minianterolateral approaches to THA are also conflicting. No randomized trials have evaluated these approaches, but comparative observational studies do exist. In a cohort of 212 patients, the mini-incision was associated with less blood loss and shorter operating time; however, postoperative blood loss and complications did not differ between groups.[19] In another study, patients with THA via a mini-incision lateral approach had significantly earlier ambulation, less transfer assistance, and more favorable discharge dispositions; they also had decreased transfusion requirements and better functional recovery with early physical therapy.[6] Other investigators have shown that THA can be performed safely through a minimal incision anterolateral approach. Early results have demonstrated an increase in the length of operation compared with a standard approach, despite selection of smaller patients, but the authors expect this result will change with further experience. No benefit has been found with respect to perioperative blood loss, but the authors' results do suggest that for patients without additional medical problems, this technique may lead to a reduction in the length of hospital stay.[7]

Minimally invasive is often equated with "small incisions." However, the length of the incision was not reported to affect outcomes (function, pain, hospital stay) in a cohort of 60 patients treated with a mini- versus standard lateral incision for THA.[8]

The Anterior Surgical Approach to THA

In contrast to the other approaches about the hip, the anterior approach is an intermuscular approach that avoids detachment of muscle from bone. The biologic rationale for a single-incision anterior approach with preservation of muscle

Table 7
Outcome data (complications)

Characteristic	n (%)
Intraoperative complications	
Greater trochanter	12
Femoral head migration	1
Perforation	2
Calcar split	10
Femur fracture	11
Excessive bleeding	1
Acetabular #	1
Posterior Column Pelvic #	1
Postoperative complications	
Cardiovascular	
Congestive heart failure	1
Stroke	1
Atrial fibrillation	1
Myocardial infarction	1
Mild hypertension	1
Postoperative tachycardia	1
Pulmonary embolism	3
Peroneal clot	1
DVT	10
Psychological	
Delerium	2
Transient confusion	1
Neurological	
Anterolateral thigh parasthesia	1
Lateral femoral cutaneous nerve palsy	7
Lateral thigh numbness	5
Musculoskeletal	
Acetabular #	4
Pelvic #	2
Strain of tensor fasica lata muscle; partial tear	1
Marked pain	9
Soft tissue strain	1
Heterotopic bone formation	7
Hip abductor weakness/ quadriceps atrophy	3
Hip bursitis	1
Spinal stenosis	1
Leg-length discrepancy	9
Femur fracture conservative management	1
Nondisplaced fracture greater trochanter	1
Wound complications	
Wound hematoma	5
Infection	10
Rash around incision	1
Stitch abscess	8
Subcutaneous hemorrhaging from a drain site	3
Genitourinary	
Urinary Retention	1
Prostate problems	1
Urinary tract infection	1
Upper gastrointestinal bleed	2
Lower gastrointestinal bleed	1
Miscellaneous	
Hypokalemia	1
Postoperative anemia	16
Medication sensitivity	2
Seroma	6
Fever	2
Severe nausea	1
Edema	8
Death	1

Patients may have had multiple complications.

insertions is strong in comparison to posterior-muscle splitting or lateral-abductor splitting approaches. While the goal is to preserve all tendon attachments, one or more of the posterior rotator tendons may require partial release to facilitate femoral canal preparation. The authors' experience suggests that the obturator internus is most often released followed by the piriformis.

Proponents of the approach do not advocate small incisions for the approach, as the focus remains on sparing tissues rather than small incisions. The authors' single-incision anterior approach using intermuscular planes allows a surgical approach to the hip and implantation of a total prosthesis with no muscle, tendon, or trochanteric section, even partially. The single-incision approach allows for adequate positioning of the two prosthetic components, and preserving the muscular potential may further contribute to dynamic stabilization of the hip.

The anterior intermuscular approach has been the subject of two large observational cohort studies.[10–13] Siguier and colleagues[10] treated 1,037 patients with the anterior approach to THA between June 1993 and June 2000. The dislocation rate was 0.96% (10 of 1,037 hips). In another study, Keggi and colleagues reported their series of 2,132 primary THAs performed via the anterior approach.[11] Keggi's study reported a dislocation rate of 1.3% and excellent early patient function.

Table 8
Functional outcome

WOMAC	Preoperative	3-Months Postoperative	6-Months Postoperative	1-Year Postoperative	2-Years Postoperative	3-Years Postoperative
			Follow-up Time Points			
WOMAC Pain score	n = 307 75.11 (19.820)	n = 32 96.62 (3.114)	n = 206 90.44 (12.177)	n = 239 91.31 (12.989)	n = 89 93.07 (8.354)	n = 16 93.31 (1.926)
WOMAC Function score	n = 306 45.27 (12.112)	n = 32 88.14 (9.888)	n = 205 83.40 (15.268)	n = 236 83.43 (14.737)	n = 88 82.02 (13.406)	n = 16 77.33 (6.477)

Whether the results of this muscle-sparing approach can be extrapolated to surgeons with less experience remains unknown.

Matta and colleagues[14] described a single surgeon series of 437 consecutive, unselected patients who had 494 primary THA surgeries done through an anterior approach on an orthopedic table from September 1996 to September 2004. Three patients sustained dislocations for an overall dislocation rate of 0.6%, and no patients required revision surgery for recurrent dislocation. There were 17 operative complications, including one deep infection, three wound infections, one transient femoral nerve palsy, three greater trochanter fractures, two femoral shaft fractures, four calcar fractures, and three ankle fractures.

Across participating surgeons in the authors' study, a dislocation rate of 0.6% (8 dislocations) was found, and 0.2% (3 dislocations) required implant revision. Analysis across surgeons did not reveal clustering of dislocations in any particular center. The current series did not identify any ankle fractures and may reflect improved learning curve in the technique.

Another important finding of the authors' study is the early return to function, which reached plateau levels by 3 months. The study was limited by few centers collecting this data and using 3 months as the first evaluation point. It remains plausible that even earlier functional gains are realized with this approach. Future studies need to evaluate function at earlier time points throughout the first year. The findings at 1 year were consistent with functional gains (WOMAC scores) reported for standard THA.[20] Knutsson and Engberg[21] evaluated quality of life (sickness-impact profile) following conventional THA. They identified significant differences in patients' total, physical, and psychosocial quality of life 6 months postoperatively compared with preoperative status, but not between the preoperative status and 6 weeks after the total hip replacement surgery.

The authors' data suggests that surgeons with greater than 100 hip cases reduce overall complication rates. While this requires confirmation in other studies evaluating this approach, these findings are not inconsistent with learning curves reported for conventional THA.[22–25] In a cohort of 57,488 Medicare beneficiaries, Katz and colleagues[23] identified a significant decrease in complications in high-volume surgeons (>100 THAs) compared with low-volume surgeons (<50 THAs).

Need for Further Research

The anterior approach is gaining popularity, largely based upon anecdotal surgeon experiences with

Table 9
Surgical experience and outcomes (learning curve)

Center	n	Number of Years of Anterior Approach Practice	Number of Complications	Number of Revision Surgeries
1	110	2	8 (7.3%)	5 (4.5%)
2	35	7	5 (14.3%)	3 (8.6%)
3	313	4	21 (6.7%)	5 (1.6%)
4	73	2	20 (27.4%)	2 (2.7%)
5	221	2	14 (6.3%)	1 (0.4%)
6	198	3	38 (19.2%)	11 (5.5%)
7	52	5	9 (17.3%)	3 (5.7%)
8	84	2	19 (22.6%)	0

the technique. Marketing has further led to patientled promotion of tissue-sparing and other less-invasive approaches to arthroplasty. Evidence-based medicine posits that health care decisions should not be based upon opinion but rather the best available research. The authors' study demonstrates that the anterior approach to THA can be performed safely by surgeons with varying experience in the approach and technique. Additional studies are required to further delineate the learning curve, factors associated with prognosis following this approach, and return-to-function in comparison with alternative surgical approaches to THA.

SUMMARY

The anterior approach THA with an orthopedic table is a safe approach, with results generalizable to surgeons with varying surgical experience. Longer term follow-up and comparative studies are needed before widespread endorsement of this surgical approach to THA.

APPENDIX 1: ATHAC INVESTIGATORS

Steering Committee: Joel M. Matta, MD (chair), Santa Monica, CA; Mohit Bhandari, MD, Hamilton, ON; David Dodgin, MD, Walnut Creek, CA.

Study Concept and Design: Mohit Bhandari, MD, Joel M. Matta, MD, Stefan Kreuzer, MD, David Dodgin, MD, Gary Bradley, MD.

Study Coordination: Mohit Bhandari, MD (chair), Sheila Sprague, MSc (senior coordinator), Natalie Sidorkiewicz (research assistant), and Tashay Mignot (research assistant).

Writing Committee: Mohit Bhandari, MD (chair), Joel M. Matta, MD, Dave Dodgin, MD, Charles Clark, Phil Kregor, MD, Gary Bradley, MD, and Lester Little, MD.

Participating Centers: Gary Bradley, MD, Santa Barbara, CA; Jim Grimes, MD, Bakersfield, CA; John Masonis, MD, Charlotte, NC; Stefan Kreuzer, MD, Houston, TX; Andrew Yun, MD, Inglewood, CA; Gary Matthys, MD, Fargo, ND; Brian Jewett, MD, Eugene, OR; Michael Bellino, MD, Palo Alto, CA, and Joel Matta, MD, Santa Monica, CA.

APPENDIX 2: INTERVENTION (ANTERIOR TECHNIQUE FOR THA)

After administration of general or regional anesthesia, the patient is placed in the supine position on the ProFX table. A perineal post is used and the feet placed in the traction boots. It is normal to use a leg support for the leg that will not be operated on and no leg support for the hip that will be operated on. The hip that will not be operated on is placed in neutral rotation, extension, and abduction-adduction to serve as a radiographic reference for the operated side. The jack that will raise and lower the femoral hook is placed near the side of the patient so that the hook bracket will lie roughly parallel to the long axis of the patient. Avoiding external rotation of the hip to be operated on will make the external landmarks of the hip more reliable and enhance the landmark of the natural bulge of the tensor fascia lata muscle. The table should be leveled with the table-level button on the hand control. It is normal for the patient's arms to be placed roughly perpendicular outward and not over the chest.

The normal team consists of the surgeon, his assistant, the anesthesiologist, the scrub nurse, circulating nurse/table operator, and the X-ray technician. The following description refers to actions that may be taken by the surgeon, his assistant, or the operator of the ProFX table.

Though the incision is normally small (8 cm to 12 cm), drape a relatively wide area from just proximal to the iliac crest to the junction of the middle and distal thirds of the thigh. Draping a relatively wide area around the incision enhances the sterility by making the vinyl skin covering less likely to detach and thereby allowing mobility of the drape edges. In addition, the wider draping allows additional extensile access, if necessary.

The normal incision starts 2-cm posterior and slightly distal to the anterior superior iliac spine. This straight incision extends in a distal and slightly posterior direction to a point 2-cm to 3-cm anterior to the greater trochanter. On thinner patients, the bulge of the tensor fascia lata muscle marks the center of the line of the incision. After incision of the skin and subcutaneous, the tensor can be seen through the translucent fascia lata. Incise the fascial lata over the tensor and continue the fascial incission slightly distal and proximal to the ends of the skin incision.

Lift the fascia lata off the medial portion of the tensor and follow the interval medial to the tensor in a posterior and proximal direction. Dissection by feel is most efficient at this point and the lateral hip capsule can be easily palpated. Place a cobra retractor along the lateral hip capsule and retract the sartorius and rectus femorus muscles medially with a Hibbs retractor. It is easy to make the mistake of perforating and incompletely retracting the gluteus minimus muscle with the cobra, so check for this. If the retractors are properly placed the reflected head of the rectus that follows the lateral acetabular rim will be visible. A small periosteal elevator placed just distal to the reflected head and directed medial and distal elevates the iliopsoas and rectus femorus muscles from the anterior capsule. The elevator opens the path for a second cobra retractor placed on the medial hip capsule.

The medial and lateral retraction of the cobras brings the lateral femoral circumflex vessels into view as they cross the distal portion of the wound. These vessels are clamped, cauterized, and transected. Further distal splitting of the aponeurosis that overlies the anterior capsule and at times excision of a fat pad enhances exposure of the capsule and the origin of the vastus lateralis muscle. A trapezoidal section of the anterior capsule (wider laterally and narrower medially) is now excised, followed by placing the tips of the cobra retractors inside the medial and lateral capsule. A release of the lateral capsule parallel to the lateral acetabular rim will facilitate dislocation. In addition, excise the capsule at the base of the antero-lateral neck to expose the anterior junction of the neck and greater trochanter. This base of the neck exposure is facilitated by a Hibbs retractor that retracts the vastus and distal tensor.

A narrow Hohman retractor is now placed on the antero-lateral acetabular rim. With this exposure the antero-lateral labrum is excised and

sometimes an associated osteophyte. Distal traction on the extremity will create a small gap between the femoral head and the roof of the acetabulum. A femoral head skid is placed into this gap and rotated to a supero-medial position. The traction is released. As the extremity and hip are externally rotated and leverage applied to the skid, the hip is dislocated anteriorly and the femur externally rotated 90°. If the hip is unusually difficult to dislocate, check for adequate capsular release and osteophyte excision and extend the hip slightly. After dislocation, place the tip of a narrow Hohman retractor distal to the lesser trochanter and beneath the vastus lateralis origin. Transect the capsule on the medial neck parallel to the neck and expose the lesser trochanter and posterior neck. During exposure of the posterior and medial neck, keep in mind that Hohman retraction of the vastus protects the innervation of this muscle, which comes from medial and at a surprisingly proximal location. Happily however, this muscle is typically also enervated more distally. Reapply traction, internally rotate, and reduce the hip.

Replace the cobra retractors around the medial and lateral neck and retract the vastus origin and distal tensor with a Hibbs. Cut the femoral neck with a reciprocating saw at the desired level and angle. Use the junction of the lateral shoulder of the neck and greater trochanter as the indicator for the level of the cut and place the lateral portion of the cut slightly distal to this point. Cut the medial portion of the neck first and take care to not cut the greater trochanter with the saw. The neck cut is completed with an osteotome placed in the sagital plane that divides the lateral neck from the medial greater trochanter. The level of the neck cut is a little more difficult to judge than from posterior. The author (MB) has experimented with cutting guides but now simply "eyeballs" the cut. Drill a 4.5-mm diameter hole into the anterior head and then insert the femoral head corkscrew. Extract the head.

The original technique of Robert Judet (still used by Theirry Judet) is to cut the neck with the hip dislocated. The level of the cut is, in this case, judged by the level of the lesser trochanter. This technique introduces some danger of continuing the cut into the greater trochanter. The cut is completed by an osteotome to the supero-lateral neck.

Begin the anterior THA by cutting the neck in situ and then extracting the head. The advantage to this technique is that it avoids the dislocation step. The disadvantage is that the head is more difficult to extract and at times the head must be sectioned to remove it. The dislocation step increases the rotational mobility of the femur and thereby enhances femoral exposure for broaching and prosthesis insertion.

Throughout the procedure the surgeon will find that the tensor fascia lata muscle is potentially vulnerable to injury. Take care not to lever too hard on this muscle with retractors. During cutting of the neck, the relatively dull side of the oscillating saw blade will cut the muscle if it contacts it. Levering the femoral head skid through wide angles can also lacerate the muscle. As the cut femoral neck is extracted, the sharp bony edge can also lacerate the muscle, so use a Rongeur to round the neck cut or at least take care to protect the muscle with the Hibbs during extraction. Attention to this muscle needs to continue during the acetabular reaming and insertion and femoral broaching phases. If an initial injury to the muscle fibers is avoided, the muscle seems to hold up well through the procedure. On the other hand, an early laceration to the surface of the tensor seems to hurt its capability to resist further damage. The ProFX table, however, makes preservation of the soft tissues easier by its external and internal control of the femur, and thereby makes leverage against the soft tissues less necessary.

The acetabulum is now visualized and prepared. External rotation of the femur of about 30° usually facilitates acetabular exposure. A trochanteric retractor is preferred over the anterior rim of the acetabulum to retract the anterior muscles. Take care to place the tip of this retractor on bone and not into the anterior soft tissues. A posterior retractor is placed with the tip initially on the postero-superior rim and subsequently on the mid-posterior rim. Excise the labrum circumferentially. Excise part of the posterior capsule that bulges over the posterior rim. Excision of the most prominent band of inferior capsule will facilitate later placement of the acetabular liner. Begin reaming under direct vision and later check with the image intensifier to confirm depth of reaming and adequate circumference. The indicators of torque and acetabular appearance are also used.

Insert the acetabular prosthesis with a normal straight inserter. The author (MB) uses the image intensifier to watch the position and progressive seating of the prosthesis. Angulate the image 5° away from the midline and 5° cephalad to simulate the direction of the X-ray beam on a postoperative AP pelvis. Before using image control, confirm that the pelvis is level with a midline image view. Symmetry of the obturator foramina or centering of the coxyx to the symphysis confirms a level pelvis. If the pelvis is not level, the table can be tilted to compensate as needed. The liner is inserted in the normal fashion and prior excision of

labrum and prominent posterior and inferior capsule will facilitate this. To shorten the distal portion of the incision, it is possible to use angulated reamers and angulated acetabular insertion devices.

The use of the image intensifier during the procedure will vary according to the surgeon's preference. It was not used by Robert Judet and is not currently used by Theirry Judet. To use it for reaming is probably most controversial. It is advocated for acetabular positioning and also to check leg length with the femoral trials. However, the procedure can be done completely without it while relying on the traditional methods of preoperative planning, guides, relation to bony or Steinman pin landmarks, as well as soft-tissue tension. Maintenance of a 1-m distance from the image makes personnel X-ray exposure unmeasurable by radiation badges.

Following acetabular insertion, the gross traction control on the table is released and the femur internally rotated to neutral. The vastus ridge is palpated and the femoral hook placed just distal to this and around the posterior femur. The hook is attached to the most convenient hole on the bracket. The femur is now externally rotated 90° and the hip hyperextended and adducted. This position is achieved by rotating the wheel at the end of the leg spar, dropping the leg spar to the floor, and adducting it. Remember to release the gross traction lock to prevent a hyperextension stretch to the femoral nerve.

For proximal femoral exposure, the author (MB) use a long-handled cobra with the tip on the posterior femoral neck (now facing medially) and place the tip of the trochanteric retractor posterior to the tip of the trochanter. It is now necessary to visualize the medial aspect of the greater trochanter and obtain some femoral mobility that allows the femur to come slightly lateral and anterior. The proximal femur is now raised by the femoral hook until the tissues come under moderate tension. It is important to feel the tension by manually lifting the hook up and down as the hook is raised. You should be able to manually lift the femur higher than the level the hook has raised it to. Too much tension can cause a fracture of the greater trochanter. Following this initial maneuver, the posterior ridge of the greater trochanter usually lies posterior to the posterior rim of the acetabulum. The femur needs to be mobile enough so that lateral and anterior displacement brings the posterior edge of the trochanter lateral and anterior to the posterior rim of the acetabulum. A band of postero-superior capsule will be seen to tether the femur at its attachment to the sulcus between the lateral neck remnant and the medial trochanter. Excise this attachment and replace the trochanteric retractor closer to the tip of the trochanter so that it retracts the gluteus minimus and medius, and possibly also the piriformis and obturator internus tendons. The obturator externus tendon insertion will be found at the point normally termed the "piriformis fossa." The piriformis and obturator internus tendons insert on the mid portion of the tip of the greater trochanter. Manually check the mobility of the femur by pulling on the hook and if it is mobile enough, raise the jack to support the femur in the desired position. Depending on the requirements for femoral mobility, the surgeon may choose to release one or more of the short external rotator tendons.

REFERENCES

1. Buckwalter JA, Saltzman C, Brown T. The impact of osteoarthritis: implications for research. Clin Orthop Relat Res 2004;427(Suppl):S6–15.

2. Ogonda L, Wilson R, Archbold P, et al. A minimal-incision technique in total hip arthroplasty does not improve early postoperative outcomes. A prospective, randomized, controlled trial. J Bone Joint Surg Am 2005;87-A:701–10.

3. Woolson ST, Mow CS, Syquia JF, et al. Comparison of primary total hip replacements performed with a standard incision or a mini-incision. J Bone Joint Surg Am 2004;86-A:1353–8.

4. Berger RA. The technique of minimally invasive total hip arthroplasty using the two-incision approach. Instr Course Lect 2004;53:149–55.

5. Irving JF. Direct two-incision total hip replacement without fluoroscopy. Orthop Clin North Am 2004;35: 173–81.

6. Wenz JF, Gurkan I, Jibodh SR. Mini-incision total hip arthroplasty: a comparative assessment of perioperative outcomes. Orthopedics 2002;25:1031–43.

7. Howell JR, Masri BA, Duncan CP. Minimally invasive versus standard incision anterolateral hip replacement: a comparative study. Orthop Clin North Am 2004;35:153–62.

8. de Beer J, Petruccelli D, Zalzal P, et al. Single-incision, minimally invasive total hip arthroplasty: length doesn't matter. J Arthroplasty 2004;19:945–50.

9. Bertin KC, Rottinger H. Anterolateral mini-incision hip replacement surgery: a modified Watson-Jones approach. Clin Orthop Relat Res 2004;429:248–55.

10. Siguier T, Siguier M, Brumpt B. Mini-incision anterior approach does not increase dislocation rate: a study of 1037 total hip replacements. Clin Orthop Relat Res 2004;426:164–73.

11. Kennon R, Keggi J, Zatorski LE, et al. Total hip arthroplasty through a minimally invasive anterior surgical approach. J Bone Joint Surg Am 2003;85-A:39–48.

12. Wright JM, Crockett HC, Delgado S, et al. Mini-incision for total hip arthroplasty: a prospective, controlled investigation with 5-year follow-up evaluation. J Arthroplasty 2004;19:538–45.

13. Kennon R, Keggi J, Zatorski LE, et al. Anterior approach for total hip arthroplasty: beyond the minimally invasive technique. J Bone Joint Surg Am 2004;86-A:91–7.

14. Matta JM, Shahrdar C, Ferguson T. Single-incision anterior approach for total hip arthroplasty on an orthopaedic table. Clin Orthop Relat Res 2005;441: 115–24.

15. Tubach F, Ravaud P, Baron G, et al. Evaluation of clinically relevant changes in patient reported outcomes in knee and hip osteoarthritis: the minimal clinically important improvement. Ann Rheum Dis 2005;64:29–33.

16. Sculco TP. Minimally invasive total hip arthroplasty: in the affirmative. J Arthroplasty 2004;19:78–80.

17. Nakamura S, Matsuda K, Arai N, et al. Mini-incision posterior approach for total hip arthroplasty. Int Orthop 2004;28:214–7. Epub 2004 May 28.

18. DiGioia AM 3rd, Plakseychuk AY, Levison TJ, et al. Mini-incision technique for total hip arthroplasty with navigation. J Arthroplasty 2003;18:123–8.

19. Higuchi F, Gotoh M, Yamaguchi N, et al. Minimally invasive uncemented total hip arthroplasty through an anterolateral approach with a shorter skin incision. J Orthop Sci 2003;8:812–7.

20. Nilsdotter AK, Lohmander LS. Patient relevant outcomes after total hip replacement. A comparison between different surgical techniques. Health Qual Life Outcomes 2003;11:21–6.

21. Knutsson S, Engberg IB. An evaluation of patients' quality of life before, 6 weeks and 6 months after total hip replacement surgery. J Adv Nurs 1999;30: 1349–59.

22. Sharkey PF, Shastri S, Teloken MA, et al. Relationship between surgical volume and early outcomes of total hip arthroplasty: do results continue to get better? J Arthroplasty 2004;19:694–9.

23. Katz JN, Phillips CB, Baron JA, et al. Association of hospital and surgeon volume of total hip replacement with functional status and satisfaction three years following surgery. Arthritis Rheum 2003;48:560–8.

24. Losina E, Barrett J, Mahomed NN, et al. Early failures of total hip replacement: effect of surgeon volume. Arthritis Rheum 2004;50:1338–43.

25. Shervin N, Rubash HE, Katz JN. Orthopaedic procedure volume and patient outcomes: a systematic literature review. Clin Orthop Relat Res 2007; 457:35–41.

Anterior-Supine Minimally Invasive Total Hip Arthroplasty: Defining the Learning Curve

Brian E. Seng, DO[a], Keith R. Berend, MD[a,b,c,*], Andrew F. Ajluni, DO[a], Adolph V. Lombardi, Jr., MD, FACS[a,b,c,d]

KEYWORDS

- Anterior-supine • Total hip arthroplasty
- Minimally invasive • Surgical approach • Muscle-sparing
- Short stems • Smith-Petersen interval
- Specialized microplasty instrumentation
- Fluoroscopic guidance

The reported advantages of minimally invasive total hip arthroplasty (THA) include less blood loss, less pain, and shorter hospital stays, all of which combine to provide a faster recovery.[1–4] A comparable number of studies, however, have failed to show any significant advantage over standard approaches.[5–8] It has been argued that these minimally invasive techniques require a significant learning curve and are associated with an increased risk of early complications.[3,9–12] Furthermore, the long-term outcomes of these minimally invasive procedures, in terms of fixation and implant longevity, remain unproven.

In this discussion the recent surgical approaches known as "minimally invasive THA" are divided into three basic categories: an abbreviated incision ("small incision"), modifications of standard approaches with smaller incisions and less soft tissue dissection ("less invasive"), and novel approaches that reportedly do not cut muscle ("minimally invasive"). The authors have a broad experience during the past 7 years with a less-invasive (LIS) modification of the direct-lateral approach (modified Hardinge). We previously have reported less blood loss and a shorter hospital stay by implementing this approach.[13] Others have argued that the LIS direct lateral approach does not provide an advantage over the traditional approach.[5] Importantly, the soft tissue dissection still requires splitting and repairing the abductor musculature.

Recently, multiple reports have detailed various techniques of minimally invasive THA performed through a single anterior incision via the Smith-Petersen interval.[4,14–16] A few early reports of this anterior approach in hip arthroplasty include those by Judet[17] and Light and Keggi,[18] the latter often incorporating multiple accessory incisions

A.V.L. and K.R.B. receive royalties and have consulting agreements with Biomet, Inc. K.R.B. has consulting agreements with Synvasive and Salient Surgical Technologies. A.V.L. receives royalties from Innomed, Inc., and is a board member of a foundation that has received support from Allergan, Biomet, GlaxoSmithKline, Medtronic, Merck, Mount Carmel New Albany Surgical Hosptial, and Smith & Nephew.

[a] Joint Implant Surgeons, Inc., 7277 Smith's Mill Road, New Albany, OH 43054, USA
[b] Mount Carmel Health System, 7333 Smith's Mill Road, New Albany, OH 43054, USA
[c] Department of Orthopaedics, The Ohio State University, 410 West 10th Avenue, Columbus, OH 43210, USA
[d] Department of Biomedical Engineering, The Ohio State University, 410 West 10th Avenue, Columbus, OH 43210, USA
* Corresponding author. Joint Implant Surgeons, Inc., 7277 Smith's Mill Road, Suite 200, New Albany, OH 43054.
E-mail address: berendkr@joint-surgeons.com (K.R. Berend).

Orthop Clin N Am 40 (2009) 343–350
doi:10.1016/j.ocl.2009.01.002

required by older style instruments. The anterior interval is both intermuscular and internervous, potentially providing the claimed advantages of little or no muscle dissection and offering a true minimally invasive alternative. These anterior-based approaches, like most other LIS or minimally invasive approaches, are aided by specialized instrumentation. One such approach is the anterior-supine intermuscular (ASI) technique using specialized microplasty (Biomet, Warsaw, IN) instrumentation.

Matta and colleagues[14] describe the use of specialized or modified operative fracture tables, similar to those used for pelvic fracture surgery. Potential disadvantages of this technique include the cost of the table, difficulty in checking range of motion and stability, and equipment-related fractures. Two reports included ankle fractures related to the use of these specialized tables that require the foot to be fixed in a foot holder.[14,15] Alternative techniques include the use of a standard radiolucent operative table with extreme hyperextension and the use of a table-mounted femoral elevator with the legs draped free.

This article examines the early learning curve for the introduction of the ASI approach in a high-volume THA practice. The authors attempt to define the learning curve, examine perioperative complications, and determine whether ASI offers and advantage in early recovery advantage compared with the LIS direct lateral approach. A detailed review of the authors' operative approach is included.

MATERIALS AND METHODS

The first ASI THA was performed at Joint Implant Surgeons, Inc., in February 2007. All primary THAs performed between January 2007 and March 2008 by a single surgeon (KRB) were examined. To obviate the long learning curve, the surgeon participated in three training sessions with a total of five cadavers and carefully selected the first patients to decrease difficulty. The initial patients selected were thin female patients with high offset and minimal deformity. Throughout the learning curve, as described later, the difficulty of cases increased. Additionally, the surgeon scheduled only one ASI THA per surgical day for the first several weeks of experience. Three categories of approaches were used: ASI, LIS, and standard direct lateral (STD). All patients were entered prospectively into our internal review board–approved clinical database and electronic medical record. The database was reviewed retrospectively for patient demographics, surgical and hospital data, and follow-up data. Patient demographics evaluated included age, gender, diagnosis, height, weight, and body mass index (BMI). Surgical data included duration (skin-to-skin operative time), estimated blood loss, and intraoperative complications. Hospital data included allogenic blood transfusions and length of stay. Follow-up data from office visits 6 weeks after surgery and any subsequent office visits included the standard variables identified with the Harris Hip Score (HHS):[19] pain, walking ability, assistive device usage, and limp. Both preoperative and postoperative Lower Extremity Activity Scale (LEAS) scores were calculated also.[20] The results of data comparing the ASI and LIS groups are provided.

The direct lateral approach used was described previously by Frndak and colleagues[21] and was performed in the lateral decubitus position. The LIS approach involved an abbreviated skin and fascial incision with a limited abductor muscle dissection compared with the standard approach. This LIS approach is performed in the lateral decubitus position and also has been previously described.[13]

The ASI approach involves the use of a standard radiolucent operative table with the table extender at the foot of the bed and the patient supine. Fluoroscopy is used in every case. The patient is positioned with the pubic symphysis at the table break for subsequent positioning during femoral preparation and implant insertion (**Fig. 1**). Both lower limbs are prepped and draped separately for positioning during surgery. The proximal end of the incision is placed approximately two finger-breadths distal and two finger-breadths lateral to the anterior-superior iliac spine (**Fig. 2**). An 8- to 10-cm incision is used. The incision is placed in this lateral position to avoid the lateral femoral cutaneous nerve. (Two-incision techniques place

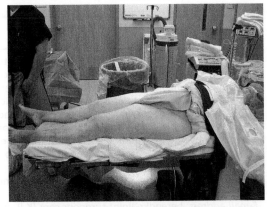

Fig. 1. Correct patient positioning with the pubic symphysis directly over the table break.

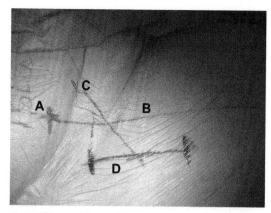

Fig. 2. Skin markings of the right hip depicting (A) the anterior superior iliac spine (ASIS), (B) a reference line drawn from the ASIS to the center of the patella, (C) the center of the femoral neck confirmed by fluoroscopy, and (D) the correct placement of the skin incision.

the anterior incision more medially.) Correct incision position is confirmed with fluoroscopy (**Fig. 3**). The fascia overlying the tensor fascia lata (TFL) muscle is split the length of the incision, and the muscle is bluntly dissected away from the interval between TFL and the sartorius muscle, with care taken to protect the fascia between the two for protection of the sartorius muscle body. The deep muscle fascia of the TFL then is split, exposing the lateral circumflex vessels. These muscles are ligated, cauterized, and transected. With blunt dissection, retractors are placed over and under the femoral neck. The inferior retractor lies under the rectus muscle and over the vastus.

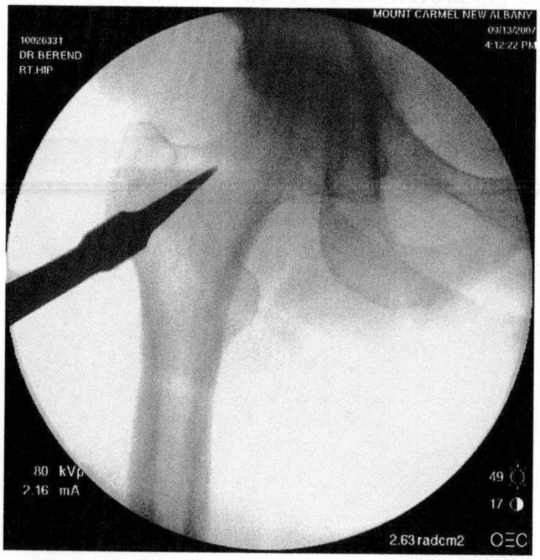

A sharp, pointed retractor then is used to peel the rectus carefully off the anterior capsule and is placed over the anterior rim of the acetabulum.

The exposed anterior capsule then is excised, exposing the femoral neck. Meticulous capsular resection at this step makes subsequent steps of acetabular preparation easier. The inferior and superior femoral neck retractors are replaced intracapsularly, and the femoral neck resection is performed based on preoperative templating and is confirmed with fluoroscopy. A subcapital resection and final neck resection are performed to create a napkin-ring of femoral neck. A threaded Steinman pin is used to remove the napkin-ring and femoral head sequentially. A sharp retractor is placed superiorly (at the 3 o'clock position on a left hip), a double-pronged posterior retractor is placed on the ischium (at approximately 7 o'clock for a left hip), and the anterior retractor is replaced if necessary. The labrum, osteophytes, and any capsule that lies in the way of acetabular preparation are removed. Sequential reaming is performed under fluoroscopic guidance if necessary (**Fig. 4**). The acetabular component then is placed, and its position is confirmed with fluoroscopy (**Fig. 5**). Screws may be placed, a liner may be inserted, or a solid metal-on-metal articulation can be used.

Femoral preparation and implant insertion require specialized positioning. The anesthesiologist must jack-knife the table by dropping the foot and placing the bed into steep Trendelenburg position. The contralateral nonoperative foot is placed on a padded Mayo stand. A table-mounted femoral elevator (Omni-Tract Surgical, St. Paul, MN) is placed on the bed, and the traction hook is placed around the proximal femur, proximal to the conjoined tendon of gluteus maximus (**Fig. 6**). Retraction is placed on the femur to tension the capsule. A retractor is placed gently,

Fig. 3. Confirmation of the center of the femoral neck with fluoroscopy.

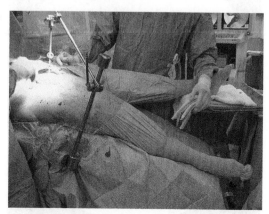

Fig. 4. Patient positioning for femoral preparation using a table-mounted femoral elevator.

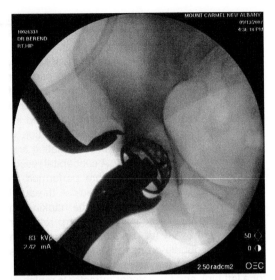

Fig. 5. Fluoroscopy image depicting acetabular reaming.

directly proximal to the greater trochanter, creating a fold of the proximal/superior capsule that can be excised easily. The trochanteric retractor then is replaced to elevate the proximal femur. The proximal/superior capsule is dissected from the trochanter from anterior to posterior. With increasing gentle retraction via the table-mounted hook, the femur is elevated. Simultaneously, the operative limb is rotated externally and adducted underneath the nonoperative leg in a lazy "figure-four" position. Extreme knee flexion tightens the rectus and makes exposure more difficult. If the inferior capsule has not been excised, it then is dissected from the femoral neck.

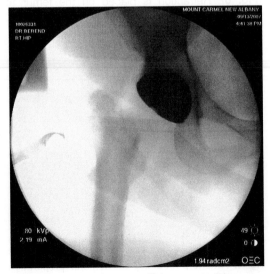

Fig. 6. Fluoroscopy image verifying cup position.

Femoral preparation then is performed. The use of a broach-only stem design is recommended because specialized offset broaches and broach handles make femoral preparation significantly easier, and direct straight reaming of the femur is difficult in most cases (**Fig. 7**). The final broach is left in place, a trial femoral neck and trial head is inserted, and the hip is relocated by releasing the traction of the table-mounted femoral elevator, internally rotating, abducting, and extending the limb. Fluoroscopic images are obtained to confirm femoral implant positioning, offset, and neck and leg length. The surgeon can measure leg length directly in the supine position through direct comparison of the medial malleoli and via fluoroscopy (**Fig. 8**).

The hip then is dislocated, and the final implant inserted. Trial reduction for leg length then can be performed, and final fluoroscopic images are obtained. The bed is returned to the flat position, the wound is irrigated, a deep drain is placed, and the wound is closed in layers. A running suture is used for the superficial tensor fascia, interrupted sutures are used subcutaneously, followed by subcutaneous running knotless suture (Quill, Angiotech, Reading, PA). The incision then is closed with skin glue (Dermabond, Ethicon, Inc, Somerville, NJ).

A standardized hospitalization and rehabilitation protocol, as previously reported, was used in all cases.[22] The protocol includes the use of pre-emptive pain and nausea medications, intrathecal spinal anesthetic and long-acting narcotic, and a periarticular soft tissue injection cocktail. This perioperative program has been reported previously, as has the authors' multimodal approach to the prevention of venous thromboembolism.[23] Patients are ambulated the day of surgery with a walker and are discharged from the hospital

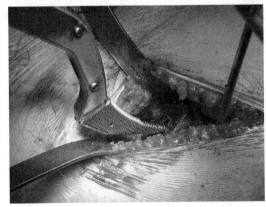

Fig. 7. Femoral preparation using an offset broach handle.

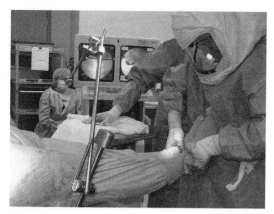

Fig. 8. Intraoperative assessment of leg length.

when they have accomplished physical therapy goals. Patients are instructed to use the walker for 2 weeks and then progress to a cane or no assistive devices when able. Routine follow-up physical and radiographic examination is performed at 6 weeks and annually thereafter.

RESULTS

Two hundred eighty-one primary THAs were performed during the study period: 22 STD (7.8%), 77 LIS (27.4%), and 182 ASI (64.8%). Throughout the study period the average operating room time was significantly longer for the ASI approach (73 minutes) than for the LIS approach (56 minutes) (*P* < .01). The average blood loss during surgery was not significantly greater for the ASI approach (162 mL) than for the LIS approach (141 mL) (*P* = .07), but the overall risk of transfusion was significantly higher in the ASI group, with 15 units of blood transfused for 182 hips compared with 1 unit transfused in 77 LSI procedures (*P*<.05).

To assess the influence of the learning curve, time intervals of 3 months were examined for changes. Fourteen percent of cases were performed via ASI in the first 3 months, 47% in the next 3 months, followed by 57%, 87%, and 89% in the subsequent three 3-month intervals. The use of the ASI procedure in more than 50% of cases (ie, in 37 cases) after 6 months indicates the surgeons' increased comfort with the procedure. The average operative time dropped significantly, from an average of 99 minutes in the first 3-month interval to 69 minutes in the third interval (*P* < .05). The average operative time over the following three intervals was 70 minutes, representing a plateau in the learning curve. The learning curve of 6 months and 37 cases coincides with this drop and subsequent plateau in operative time. The average operative time in the LIS group

was 56 minutes and remained constant throughout the study period. The average intraoperative blood loss also dropped significantly from the first 3 months to the last 3 months (*P* < .05). Interestingly, the rate of transfusions did not drop commensurate with the reduced intraoperative blood loss. A drain was used in the ASI group, and postoperative output was not tracked; no drain was used in the LIS group.

Despite a clear bias toward implementing the ASI in easier cases during the early experience, there was no difference between the ASI and the LIS groups in the average height, weight, or BMI. The average length of hospital stay was shorter for the ASI group, but not significantly so (1.9 days versus 2.0 days; *P* > .1). The average 6-week HHS was significantly higher for the ASI group than for the LIS group (81 versus 75; *P* < .0001). Despite the absence of a significant difference in the preoperative LEAS, the score was significantly higher at 6 weeks after surgery for the ASI group (8.7 versus 7.5; *P* = .01), demonstrating that the ASI procedure afforded a faster return to function and daily activities.

There were four intraoperative complications in the ASI group, all identified and corrected during the procedure. Two intraoperative proximal femoral perforations occurred, in patients number 18 and 36. These perforations occurred during stem preparation, were noted intraoperatively, and did not alter the surgical procedure. One acetabular component dislodged and required acute revision to a modular device with screws, and one intraoperative pelvic fracture occurred during cup insertion requiring bone grafting with autograft femoral head and use of a porous metal revision acetabular component.

There have been four reoperations in the ASI group: two periprosthetic fractures (at 6 weeks and 3 months), each requiring revision and cerclage cable fixation, and two wound complications requiring superficial debridement and irrigation with primary wound closure. No other reoperations have occurred, and there have been no deep infections. In the LIS group, there were three reoperations: one acute acetabular revision, and two hematomas requiring deep washout and closure over drains.

Other notable complications in the ASI group include two lateral femoral cutaneous nerve (LFCN) paresthesias, both of which resolved. There were no dislocations, femoral nerve injuries, or any clinically evident deep vein thrombosis. The overall rate of complications in the ASI group was 5.4% (10/182). None of the four intraoperative complications resulted in significant clinical problems, both LFCN paresthesias resolved, and thus the overall rate of significant clinical complications for the ASI group was 2.2% (4/182). The LIS group included one patient who had paresthesia of the lateral thigh and one who had paresthesia related to the sciatic nerve. There were three clinically evident deep vein thromboses in the LIS group, although this incidence was not found to be statistically significant. The overall rate of complications in the LIS group was 10.4% (8/77). Again, the paresthesias resolved, thus, the rate of clinically significant complications in the LIS group was 7.8% (6/77).

DISCUSSION

This study assessed the learning curve for a high-volume total joint surgeon implementing a new surgical approach into practice. After 6 months and 37 cases, more than 50% of all primary total joint arthroplasties were performed comfortably by the anterior-supine intermuscular technique. Coinciding with this time period was a drop and then a plateau in operating time and intraoperative blood loss. Although not significant, the reported intraoperative complications, specifically two proximal femoral perforations, are noted. The authors believe that exposure for preparation of the femur is technique dependent and is an early concern when learning the ASI approach. Both perforations occurred in muscular male patients who had relatively short, varus femoral neck anatomy. Sariali and colleagues[24] reported seven false reamings of the proximal femur, all noted intraoperatively and without consequence. They also noted increased difficulty in femoral exposure as an explanation.

The concept of preserving muscles and tendons is intuitively the least invasive surgical approach that in theory should lead to more rapid recovery. In the authors' study, both the 6-week HHS and the LEAS were significantly higher than in the direct lateral LIS group. This experience is in contrast to that of Kim and colleagues[12] and Ogonda and colleagues,[7] who failed to show improvement in the 6-week HHS using a mini-posterior incision, perhaps because their approach involved direct muscle transection, and identifies a difference between a small-incision approach and a truly muscle-sparing approach such as the ASI.

Often reported as a minimally invasive technique, the two-incision approach involves a modified Smith-Petersen anterior approach for insertion of the acetabular component and a supplemental posterior incision for insertion of the femoral component. This approach has allowed same-day surgery, extremely rapid recovery, and dramatic results in some surgeons' hands.[3] Interpreting the impact of the minimally invasive approach on outcomes and recovery is difficult, however, because of the concurrent implementation of an accelerated hospital pathway. In the authors' study, using identical pre-emptive anesthetic and rehabilitation techniques, they note a significantly improved early recovery using the ASI approach compared with the LIS. Additionally, cadaveric studies suggest greater muscle damage occurs with the two-incision technique than with the Smith-Petersen approach, again reinforcing the benefit of a true muscle-sparing technique.[25,26]

The intriguing question remains, what is the learning curve? Although the authors report 37 cases for their use of the ASI, a variety of other reports exist in the literature. Mears[2] reported a learning curve of 10 cases with regards to complications. Archibeck and colleagues[10] reported increased proficiency as indicated by decreased operative time and fluoroscopy use in the first 10 cases, but they also found no decrease in complications as a function of case number over the first 10 cases. They did note that surgeon experience, defined as more than 50 THAs per year, had an effect on decreased complications. Berger[3] reported performing more 40 cadaveric procedures before using the two-incision technique in his first patient, and this experience should be viewed a significant portion of any learning curve. Asayama and colleagues,[5] using a LIS direct lateral approach, reported technique-related intraoperative complications with patients number 29 and 47 during a period in which they considered themselves to be experienced in the approach. Meanwhile Woolson and colleagues[6] reported intraoperative complications among three high-volume fellowship-trained joint surgeons after they had performed 5 to 15 surgeries using the mini-posterior approach. Instances that the authors considered approach-related complications (femoral perforations) occurred during what they found to be a learning curve of 37 cases, and since then they have avoided such complications. An acetabular complication similar to those encountered intraoperatively in the ASI group also occurred in one patient in the LIS group, although it was not recognized intraoperatively and was not considered to be approach related.

Another concern is dislocation, because compromised stability puts the patient at risk of potential reoperations. One review of the literature found reported rates of dislocation ranging from 1% to 9%,[24] but the literature supports a decreased dislocation rate in cases using the anterior approach. Siguier and colleagues[15] reported a 0.96% dislocation rate using a 22-mm head in 1037 hip arthroplasties, Kennon and colleagues[4] reported a 1.3% dislocation rate in 2132 cases, and Matta and colleagues[14] reported a 0.61% incidence. Sariali and colleagues[24] reported a 1.5% rate, but further analysis showed a 2% rate with 22-mm heads and a 0.5% rate with 28-mm heads. The authors of this article did not find any early dislocations in their series.

SUMMARY

The ASI approach seems to be safe, without a dramatically high complication rate. The learning curve seems to be around 40 cases or 6 months in a high volume hip arthroplasty center, after which blood loss and operating room time stabilize, approach-related complications can be avoided, and use of the approach in the practice may be more than 50%. The early recovery of patients undergoing ASI THA is more rapid that that of patients in whom the LIS directlateral approach is used, as shown by improved 6-week HHS and LEAS. Although there were complications associated with implementing this approach, they did not occur at a significantly higher rate than with the LIS directlateral approach. Furthermore, no significant long-term sequelae were noted from the intraoperative complications. The authors suggest cadaveric training, one-on-one mentoring, and a conservative strategy for implementing ASI into a surgeon's practice. Although some surgeons may argue that the anterior approach is suitable in all cases, the authors of this article recommend against this approach in morbidly obese patients in whom the pannus of the stomach may hang over the incision, in patients who have severe proximal femoral deformity, and in some patients who have had significant previous hip surgery, because these factors certainly increase the difficulty of the operation and may obviate the recovery benefits. Although the transfusion rate seems to be higher and was not reduced even after the initial learning curve, the increased rate may be related to the use of a drain in the ASI group or an actual increase in blood loss during and after surgery. For this reason, the authors are exploring blood salvage, preoperative erythropoietin, and other methods to avoid transfusions in these patients.

REFERENCES

1. Chimento GF, Pavone V, Sharrock N, et al. Minimally invasive total hip arthroplasty. J Arthroplasty 2005; 20:139–44.

2. Berry DJ, Berger RA, Callaghan JJ, et al. Symposium: minimally invasive total hip arthroplasty. Development, early results and a critical analysis. J Bone Joint Surg Am 2003;85:2235–46.

3. Berger RA. Total hip arthroplasty using the minimally invasive two-incision approach. Clin Orthop 2003; 417:232–41.

4. Kennon RE, Keggi JM, Wetmore RS, et al. Total hip arthroplasty through a minimally invasive anterior surgical approach. J Bone Joint Surg Am 2003; 85(suppl 4):39–48.

5. Asayama I, Kinsey TL, Mahoney OM. Two-year experience using a limited-incision direct lateral approach in total hip arthroplasty. J Arthroplasty 2006;21:1083–91.

6. Woolson ST, Mow CS, Syquia JF, et al. Comparison of primary total hip replacement performed with a standard incision or a mini-incision. J Bone Joint Surg Am 2004;86:1353–8.

7. Ogonda L, Wilson R, Archbold P, et al. A minimal-incision technique in total hip arthroplasty does not improve early postoperative outcomes. J Bone Joint Surg Am 2005;87:701–10.

8. Pagnano MW, Leone J, Lewalle DG, et al. Two-incision THA had modest outcomes and some substantial complications. Clin Orthop 2005;441:86–90.

9. Bal BS, Haltom D, Aleto T, et al. Early complications of primary total hip replacement performed with a two-incision minimally invasive technique. J Bone Joint Surg Am 2005;87:2432–8.

10. Archibeck MJ, White RE Jr. Learning curve for the two-incision total hip replacement. Clin Orthop 2004;429:232–8.

11. Fehring TK, Mason JB. Catastrophic complications of minimally invasive hip surgery. A series of three cases. J Bone Joint Surg Am 2005;87:711–4.

12. Kim YH. Comparison of primary total hip arthroplasties performed with a minimally invasive technique or standard technique. J Arthroplasty 2006;21:1092–8.

13. Berend KR, Lombardi AV Jr. Total hip arthroplasty via the less invasive anterolateral abductor splitting approach. Semin Arthroplasty 2004;15:87–93.

14. Matta JM, Shahrdar C, Ferguson T. Single-incision anterior approach for total hip arthroplasty on an orthopaedic table. Clin Orthop 2005;441:115–24.

15. Siguier T, Siguier M, Brumpt B. Mini-incision anterior approach does not increase dislocation rate. Clin Orthop 2004;426:164–73.

16. Nakata K, Nishikawa M, Yamamoto K, et al. A clinical comparative study of the direct anterior with miniposterior approach. J Arthroplasty 2008 Jun 12. Epub ahead of print.

17. Judet J, Judet R. The use of an artificial femoral head for arthroplasty of the hip joint. J Bone Joint Surg Am 1950;32B:166–73.

18. Light TR, Keggi KJ. Anterior approach to hip arthroplasty. Clin Orthop 1980;152:255–60.

19. Harris WH. Traumatic arthritis of the hip after dislocation and acetabular fractures: treatment by mold arthroplasty. An end-result study using a new method of result evaluation. J Bone Joint Surg Am 1969; 51(4):737–55.

20. Saleh KJ, Mulhall KJ, Bershadsky B, et al. Development and validation of a lower-extremity activity scale. J Bone Joint Surg Am 2005;87:1985–94.

21. Frndak PA, Mallory TH, Lombardi AV Jr. Translateral surgical approach to the hip. The abductor muscle split. Clin Orthop 1993;295:135–41.

22. Berend KR, Lombardi AV Jr, Mallory TH. Rapid recovery protocol for peri-operative care of total hip and total knee arthroplasty patients. Surg Technol Int 2004;13:239–47.

23. Berend KR, Lombardi AV Jr. Multimodal venous thromboembolic disease prevention for patients undergoing primary or revision total joint arthroplasty: the role of aspirin. Am J Orthop 2006;35(1):24–9.

24. Sariali E, Leonard P, Mamoudy P. Dislocation after total hip arthroplasty using Hueter anterior approach. J Arthroplasty 2008;23:266–72.

25. Mardones R, Pagnano MW, Nemanish JP, et al. Muscle damage after total hip arthroplasty done with the two-incision and min-posterior techniques. Clin Orthop 2005;441:63–7.

26. Meneghini RM, Pagnano MW, Trousdale RT, et al. Muscle damage during MIS total hip arthroplasty Smith-Petersen versus posterior approach. Clin Orthop 2005;453:292–8.

Simultaneous Bilateral Supine Anterior Approach Total Hip Arthroplasty: Evaluation of Early Complications and Short-Term Rehabilitation

Nicholas H. Mast, MD*, Michelle Muñoz, BA, Joel Matta, MD

KEYWORDS

- Simultaneous bilateral THA • THR • Hip arthroplasty
- Anterior approach

Simultaneous bilateral total hip arthroplasty (THA) has been widely described in the orthopedic literature, but little consensus exists regarding its safety, risk, cost, and outcome. Advocates of the procedure cite a single exposure to anesthesia, improved recovery time, and decreased cost.[1–11] Opponents of the procedure cite higher risks of thrombophlebitis and of heterotopic ossification, higher transfusion requirements, higher rates of re-operation, and unacceptably high rates of transfer to rehabilitation or nursing facilities.[4,7,12–16] Previous studies have reported on these risks as they relate to simultaneous versus staged bilateral THA using the lateral decubitus position and either anterolateral or posterior approaches.

The senior author has used the supine anterior approach arthroplasty on the orthopedic table for more than 12 years. Published data from this series of patients have shown a very low dislocation rate and a very early return to unassisted ambulation.[17] An additional benefit of the supine positioning is improved access to both hips; making simultaneous bilateral procedures more manageable. Here the authors present their series of 147 simultaneous bilateral THAs with a minimum follow up of 3 months with respect to perioperative complications, cost, and return to independent function.

MATERIALS AND METHODS

The senior author prospectively gathered a series of patients undergoing THA from May 1995 to September 2007. From this database, 147 simultaneous anterior bilateral THA procedures were identified representing 294 hips. The number of simultaneous bilateral THAs performed represents approximately 10% of the authors' entire THA practice.

All patients had bilateral hip pain unresponsive to medical management and expressed interest in simultaneous bilateral THA. Perioperative medical management was performed by a single group of medical internists who preoperatively evaluated the patient. The decision to proceed with unilateral or bilateral procedures was based on surgical indication. No patients were barred from having bilateral procedures as opposed to unilateral procedures solely upon preoperative medical fitness.

The Hip and Pelvis Institute, St. John's Health Center, 2001 Santa Monica Boulevard, Suite 1090, Santa Monica, CA, 90404, USA
* Corresponding author.
E-mail address: doctormast@yahoo.com (N.H. Mast).

Orthop Clin N Am 40 (2009) 351–356
doi:10.1016/j.ocl.2009.04.002

All procedures were performed by or under the direct supervision of the senior author. As described in previous publications,[17,18] THA was performed through an anterior Hueter approach on the orthopedic table. The patient was in the supine position, and a single preoperative prep and draping was performed encompassing both hips (**Fig. 1**). THA typically was performed on the more symptomatic side first. Upon completion of this procedure and closure of the wound, THA was begun on the contralateral side.

For all procedures a single instrument set-up was used. Implants used included cemented and cementless designs as detailed in **Table 1**. Cell Saver was available for all cases. Fluoroscopic guidance was used intraoperatively to restore anatomy and leg length equality and to ensure appropriate positioning of components. Intraoperative monitoring was performed as per routine THA at the discretion of the anesthesia team.

Although slight changes have been introduced to the postoperative routine over time, the postoperative care of all patients was similar. All patients were managed with full weight-bearing therapy beginning the day of surgery or the first postoperative day. Patients were encouraged to discard walking aides when they felt comfortable doing so. Discharge was dictated by progress with therapy and when therapy goals had been met. Outpatient physical therapy was not routinely prescribed. Postoperative anticoagulation was routine and either with Coumadin or aspirin upon discharge.

All patients were evaluated in follow-up at 6 weeks following the procedure and annually thereafter. Complications were documented, and additional data were gathered with respect to date of walking without assistive device,

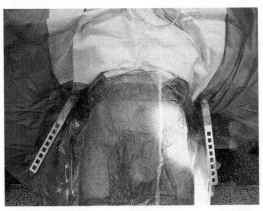

Fig. 1. For simultaneous bilateral anterior approach total hip replacement, supine positioning facilitates access to both hips. This figure shows the preoperative set-up.

postoperative complications, and functional status. Postoperative radiographs were obtained to evaluate implant appearance and position.

Data collected from perioperative records included preoperative variables such as diagnosis, preoperative pain and functional status, sex, age, and body mass index (BMI). Intraoperative variables including implant design, use of cement, operative time, blood loss, and complications such as fracture, thromboembolic disease, nerve palsy, hematoma, and early postoperative infection were identified and documented. Postoperative variables such as length of stay, disposition (home, inpatient rehabilitation, skilled nursing center stay), time to walking without an assistive device, follow-up pain scores, and function were documented.

To obtain cost data for the procedures, a subset was created that consisted of the last 10 sequential patients undergoing simultaneous anterior THA. The last 10 sequential patients were chosen to ensure that the rehabilitation protocols were standardized and that the implants used were the standard implants currently used by the authors in unilateral THA, thereby allowing a comparison with the patient population undergoing unilateral THA. Surgical and hospital charges were collected. A mean total hospital cost was created. Reimbursement was estimated based upon 2007 Medicare rates.

RESULTS

From May 1995 through September 2007, 147 simultaneous bilateral THA procedures were performed representing 294 hips. The number of simultaneous bilateral THAs performed represents 10% of the authors' entire THA practice. The mean length of follow-up for this series of patients was 4.82 years with a range of 6 months to 12.5 years. The data include nearly equal numbers of men and women, 71 and 76 respectively. Average age was 62 years with a range of 19 to 84 years. The average BMI was 27 with a range of 15 to 47.

A variety of implants were used successfully in this study (**Box 1**). Cemented and uncemented designs were implemented on the femoral side. Uncemented implant designs were used on the acetabular side. To date, no implants have required revision. By radiography, there has been no significant wear, loosening, or osteolysis noted at the time of the most recent follow-up radiograph. No patient has developed greater than Brooker grade I heterotopic ossification.

Operative data were reviewed. Operative time averaged 1.14 hours per hip (range 0.66–2.33 hours). Mean blood loss per operative side

Table 1
Demographic data for simultaneous bilateral 1° total hip arthroplasty[a]

Patient Data	Female (n = 76)		Male (n = 71)	
	Mean	Median	Mode	Range
Age	62	61	46	19–84 years
Hospital stay	4	4	3	2–14 days
Operative time	1.14	1.1	1	0.66–2.33 hours
Blood loss	289	250	200	50–900 cm³
Days to ambulation	17	14	14	1–60 days
Days without aupport	28	27	42	2–63 days
Body mass index	27	26	24	15–47

[a] Number of patients = 147; number of hips = 294.

measured 289 mL (range 50–900 mL). Cell Saver was used in all cases, and when possible this blood was returned to the patient. Thirty-nine patients (26%) committed 1 to 2 units autologous blood within 4 weeks before the procedure. Each of these patients received their banked blood postoperatively with an average postoperative autologous transfusion requirement of 1.81 units. Three of these patients required 1 to 2 additional units of allogenic blood. Of the patients not banking blood preoperatively, 18 (12%) required allogenic blood. The average transfusion requirement in these patients was 1.64 units.

Intraoperative and postoperative adverse events are summarized in **Box 2**. The most common adverse event was a postoperative anemia defined as a hemoglobin less than 10 g/dL, occurring in 27 (18%) of patients. Demographic data such as BMI, age, or gender were not predictive of postoperative anemia requiring transfusion. Postoperative ICU admissions that were not planned were noted as adverse events. Fourteen patients (9.5%) were admitted to the ICU postoperatively because of comorbidities, blood loss, or for further monitoring. Nearly all patients transferred out of the ICU on the following day. Only two patients required in the ICU for more than 1 day.

There were four direct surgical complications in this series: one femoral nerve palsy with full motor recovery by 1 year, one dislocation managed with closed reduction, one calcar crack managed with observation, and one calcar crack that went on to periprosthetic fracture. This last complication was managed successfully with open reduction and internal fixation using cable fixation. No deep infections were noted. No recurrent dislocations were noted.

Functional recovery and inpatient stays demonstrated a rather quick recovery and return to unassisted ambulation. Average inpatient hospital stay was 4 days with a range of 2 to 14 days. One hundred five patients (73%) could be discharged directly to home. The average age of those discharged to home was 60 years. The average age of the patients discharged to inpatient rehabilitation was 69 years. This difference was statistically significant ($P<.01$). Forty percent (13/33) of patients older than 70 years were discharged to inpatient rehabilitation. Interestingly, the difference in BMI was statistically significant ($P=.02$) between groups: the average BMI of those discharged to home was 26 and of those discharged to rehabilitation was 28. This difference, however, was not thought to be clinically significant.

Early clinical benefit was apparent in this patient population. By 17 days postoperatively, 57.1% of patients were able to discard assistive devices for ambulation (range, 1–60 days). By 28 days more than half (50.3%) of the patients discontinued the use of assistive devices altogether (range, 2–63 days).

One hundred twenty-four patients were followed for longer than 1 year. No failures or revisions were noted in any patients. Pain and function were scored annually. The average Merle d'Aubigne score was 17.46 at 1-year follow-up, with a range of 16 to 18.

The calculation of mean hospital costs was based on the last consecutive 10 patients. The cost per patient for simultaneous bilateral THA was $30,563, approximately $7000 more than the mean cost for a unilateral THA. These figures represent institutional operating expenses, labor, equipment, and supplies. Implant costs were standardized between the unilateral and bilateral groups. Medicare reimbursement for simultaneous bilateral THA in 2007 was $18,125.

Box 1
Surgical data

Blood loss (average): 289 cm^3

Blood loss (range (per hip): 50–900 cm^3

Cumulative transfusions

    # Autologous patients/average units: 39 patients/1.81 units

    # Homologous patients/average units (packed red blood cells, red blood cells, transfusion): 18 patients/1.64 units

Operative time (average per hip): 1.14 hours.

Operative time (range per hip): 0.66–2.33 hours.

Implants used

    Cementless femoral

        Accolade: 6

        Biomet: 2

        Corail: 192

        Zweimuller: 78

    Cementless acetabular

        Biomet: 2

        Converge: 86

        Duraloc: 12

        Pinnacle: 182

        Trident: 6

        Trilogy: 6

    Cemented femoral:

        Sulzer ms-30: 16

Box 2
Complications and recovery

Cumulative complications

Anemia (Hb < 10 g/dL): 27 patients

Dislocations: 1 patient

Infections: 0

Hematomas: 0

Unplanned ICU stays: 14 patients (average days in ICU: 1.14)

Deep vein thromboses: 0

Pulmonary embolisms: 0

Vascular: 0

Deaths: 0

Other

1 calcar crack

1 femoral fracture

1 femoral nerve palsy

Disposition

Hospital stay (average): 4 days

Hospital stay (range): 2–14 days

Discharged to home: 105 patients

Discharged to rehabilitation/skilled nursing facility/extended care facility: 27 patients

Omitted or no record: 15 patients

Days to ambulation: 17 days

Days to ambulation without assistive devices: 28 days

DISCUSSION

To date, there has only been one other review of patients undergoing simultaneous bilateral anterior approach arthroplasty. Weinstein and colleagues[19] demonstrated favorable results in a population of 43 patients older than 75 years of age. The present study aimed to expand upon this investigation by evaluating safety and early recovery in a larger patient population. A second goal of the study was to evaluate whether the anterior approach conferred any cost benefit to the hospital.

The population of patients examined by this study was an unselected consecutive series of patients who had symptomatic bilateral hip disease. Age and demographic information in this patient population were similar to previous reported series. Previous studies selected patients that were suitably "fit" for bilateral as opposed to staged procedures based on criteria such as age and medical comorbidities.[3,10–12,16,17] In this study, by contrast, the same selection criteria was used for unilateral and bilateral procedures. The surgical procedure selected was based upon orthopedic indication. The ability to change surgical preoperative clearance requirements for the procedure is felt to be directly related to supine positioning and the resultant improved monitoring and care of the patient by anesthesia.

Previous studies have demonstrated that the advantages of the supine anterior approach in THA include a low rate of dislocations and an early return to unassisted ambulation.[17,18] Similar findings have been demonstrated in this series of patients undergoing simultaneous bilateral THA. One hundred five patients (72%) could be discharged to home after a rather short inpatient stay (4 days; range, 2–14 days). Fifteen (10%) patients could be discharged to home after a 2-day inpatient stay. Similarly, early rehabilitation goals were met quickly, as evidenced by the quick return to unassisted ambulation. Relatively few patients in this series required care in an inpatient rehabilitation setting, although those over the age of 70 years might have had more difficulty with early recovery.

Simultaneous bilateral THA has received mixed reviews in orthopedic literature. Complications rates have been highly variable among series, ranging from 4.7% to 17% of cases.[1–3,6–9,11–13,15,16,20] The major complications cited include a higher risk of thrombophlebitis, heterotopic ossification, higher transfusion requirements, higher rate of reoperation, and unacceptably high rates of transfer to rehabilitation or nursing facilities.[4,7,12–16] The variation seen in complication rates reported in the literature probably is multifactorial. Studies of bilateral procedures may over- or underreport complications because of differences in study design and in the variables examined. Furthermore, a wide variety of techniques are used in simultaneous bilateral THA. Technical factors such as surgical approach, prosthesis design, and evolving postoperative protocols might contribute to the variations in complication rates and in rates of early recovery reported in the literature.

Based on previous studies,[13] the authors do not expect the long-term survivorship of their simultaneous anterior approach bilateral THA to differ from that of THA using their unilateral anterior approach. Furthermore, they expect the accuracy of component placement achieved with their technique of anterior approach THA to improve long-term outcome, dislocation rates, and wear characteristics.[18] Longer-term follow-up is necessary to support these hypotheses.

The current study focused on safety and early recovery. With respect to safety, no complication described in this series could be directly attributed to this technique alone. The rate of complications in this series certainly is within the acceptable limits for simultaneous bilateral procedures published elsewhere.[1–3,6–9,11–13,15,16,20] With respect to early recovery, this series of patients showed a very short inpatient hospital stay, a high percentage of discharge to home, and an early return to functional independence.

The authors' experience demonstrates that the simultaneous bilateral THA continues to improve from the standpoints of safety, early recovery, and rehabilitation. These findings have enormous implications with respect to the overall economic cost of the procedure. Numerous authors have documented the benefit to the health care system realized by simultaneous THA procedures.[12,21–23] Berend, and colleagues[12] investigated the financial burden carried by the hospital system and the physician in performing simultaneous versus staged arthroplasty procedures. The present findings similarly demonstrate that the hospital and surgeon bear the burden of financing this benefit. Both the hospital and surgeon lose a significant amount of potential reimbursement by performing bilateral THA as a simultaneous rather than a staged procedure. In the context of the relatively short hospital stays and early return to function seen in this study, however, the authors believe the anterior approach offers significant economic advantages to the health care system as compared with alternative surgical approaches.

SUMMARY

Simultaneous bilateral anterior approach THA has been a successful procedure with high patient demand and good short-term clinical results. Complication rates are acceptable and compare favorably with previously published series. The anterior approach takes advantage of supine positioning, allowing improved intraoperative monitoring and anesthesia care. Short-term rehabilitation goals are met early with this technique. Despite these advantages, providing this entails a large financial burden carried by the hospital and surgeon.

REFERENCES

1. Alfaro-Adrian J, Bayona F, Rech JA, et al. One- or two-stage bilateral total hip replacement. J Arthroplasty 1999;14(4):439–45.
2. Bhan S, Pankaj A, Malhotra R. One- or two-stage bilateral total hip arthroplasty: a prospective, randomised, controlled study in an Asian population. J Bone Joint Surg Br 2006;88(3):298–303.
3. Eggli S, Huckell CB, Ganz R. Bilateral total hip arthroplasty: one stage versus two stage procedure. Clin Orthop Relat Res 1996;328:108–18.
4. Huotari K, Lyytikainen O, Seitsalo S. Patient outcomes after simultaneous bilateral total hip and knee joint replacements. J Hosp Infect 2007;65(3):219–25.
5. Kim YH. Comparison of primary total hip arthroplasties performed with a minimally invasive technique or a standard technique: a prospective and randomized study. J Arthroplasty 2006;21(8):1092–8.
6. Laursen JO, Husted H, Mossing NB. One-stage bilateral total hip arthroplasty a simultaneous procedure in 79 patients. Acta Orthop Belg 2000;66(3):265–71.
7. Parvizi J, Pour AE, Peak EL, et al. One-stage bilateral total hip arthroplasty compared with unilateral total hip arthroplasty: a prospective study. J Arthroplasty 2006;21(6 Suppl 2):26–31.

8. Parvizi J, Tarity TD, Sheikh E, et al. Bilateral total hip arthroplasty: one-stage versus two-stage procedures. Clin Orthop Relat Res 2006;453:137–41.

9. Salvati EA, Hughes P, Lachiewicz P. Bilateral total hip-replacement arthroplasty in one stage. J Bone Joint Surg Am 1978;60(5):640–4.

10. Tarity TD, Herz AL, Parvizi J, et al. Ninety-day mortality after hip arthroplasty: a comparison between unilateral and simultaneous bilateral procedures. J Arthroplasty 2006;21(6 Suppl 2):60–4.

11. Welters H, Jansen I, Simon JP, et al. One-stage bilateral total hip replacement: a retrospective study of 70 patients. Acta Orthop Belg 2002; 68(3):235–41.

12. Berend KR, Lombardi AV Jr, Adams JB. Simultaneous vs staged cementless bilateral total hip arthroplasty: perioperative risk comparison. J Arthroplasty 2007; 22(6 Suppl 2):111–5.

13. Berend ME, Ritter MA, Harty LD, et al. Simultaneous bilateral versus unilateral total hip arthroplasty an outcomes analysis. J Arthroplasty 2005;20(4):421–6.

14. Macaulay W, Salvati EA, Sculco TP, et al. Single-stage bilateral total hip arthroplasty. J Am Acad Orthop Surg 2002;10(3):217–21.

15. Ritter MA, Randolph JC. Bilateral total hip arthroplasty: a simultaneous procedure. Acta Orthop Scand 1976;47(2):203–8.

16. Ritter MA, Stringer EA. Bilateral total hip arthroplasty: a single procedure. Clin Orthop Relat Res 1980;149:185–90.

17. Matta JM, Shahrdar C, Ferguson T. Single-incision anterior approach for total hip arthroplasty on an orthopaedic table. Clin Orthop Relat Res 2005;441: 115–24.

18. Matta JM, Ferguson TA. The anterior approach for hip replacement. Orthopedics 2005;28(9):927–8.

19. Weinstein MA, Keggi JM, Zatorski LE, et al. One-stage bilateral total hip arthroplasty in patients > or = 75 years. Orthopedics 2002;25(2):153–6.

20. Bracy D, Wroblewski BM. Bilateral Charnley arthroplasty as a single procedure. A report on 400 patients. J Bone Joint Surg Br 1981;63(3):354–6.

21. Lorenze M, Huo MH, Zatorski LE, et al. A comparison of the cost effectiveness of one-stage versus two-stage bilateral total hip replacement. Orthopedics 1998;21(12):1249–52.

22. Reuben JD, Meyers SJ, Cox DD, et al. Cost comparison between bilateral simultaneous, staged, and unilateral total joint arthroplasty. J Arthroplasty 1998;13(2):172–9.

23. Della Valle CJ, Idjadi J, Hiebert RN, et al. The impact of medicare reimbursement policies on simultaneous bilateral total hip and knee arthroplasty. J Arthroplasty 2003;18(1):29–34.

Hueter Anterior Approach for Hip Resurfacing: Assessment of the Learning Curve

Benoit Benoit, MD, FRCSC[a], Wade Gofton, MD, MEd, FRCSC[b],
Paul E. Beaulé, MD, FRCSC[b],*

KEYWORDS

- Hueter • Anterior approach • Hip resurfacing
- Metal on metal • Learning curve

The optimal approach for hip resurfacing arthroplasty (HRA) is controversial in respect to preservation of femoral head vascularity and the soft tissue envelope.[1] The majority of current generation metal-on-metal HRA procedures are performed through an extensile posterior approach to ensure proper component placement. In recent years, there have been significant efforts directed toward shortening hospital stay and recovery times after primary total hip replacement through multimodal pain management and surgical approaches that minimize soft tissue trauma.[2,3] Although several approaches have been advocated as less invasive, recent studies[3] have demonstrated that a mini-posterior or anterior Hueter hip resurfacing (HHR) approach can minimize the recovery time of patients undergoing primary total hip replacement.[4,5]

However, approaches favoring smaller incisions can increase the risk of component malposition or even lead to catastrophic complications.[6] This is especially relevant to HRA where poor implant position can lead to premature failure[7,8] and increased release of metal debris.[9,10] One key aspect to any surgical approach for implantation of a hip prosthesis is proper visualization for bony preparation and respect of anatomic planes for dissection. The HHR approach provides this opportunity through internervous dissection between femoral nerve (psoas and rectus femoris) and superior gluteal nerve (tensor and gluteus medius and minimus)[11] and through preservation of the soft tissue envelope and blood supply to the femoral head.[12] The purpose of this article is to evaluate the safety and the learning curve with the less invasive Hueter approach in performing hip resurfacing.

MATERIAL AND METHODS

One hundred patients who underwent metal-on-metal hip resurfacing with a minimum follow-up of 6 months were reviewed. The first 50 hip resurfacings performed with a HHR approach were compared with the last fifty consecutive primary hip resurfacing done using the surgical dislocation approach (SDA) of Ganz and colleagues.[13] The mean age of the group was 47.8 years (HHR 48.6; SDA 47.2, $P = .353$). There were 85 males and 15 females (HHR 44:6 male/female; SDA 41:9 male/female, $P = .122$). Baseline demographic and clinical data are presented in **Table 1**. The majority of patients in both groups had osteoarthritis, with the remainder having inflammatory arthritis, osteonecrosis, and low-grade developmental dysplasia of the hip or posttraumatic arthritis. This was a consecutive patient

[a] Chirurgien orthopédique, Hôpital Sacré-Coeur de Montréal, Université de Montréal, 3980 Berri, Montréal, Québec, H2L 4H1, Canada
[b] Adult Reconstruction Service, The Ottawa Hospital, University of Ottawa, 501 Smyth Road CCW 1646, Ottawa, Ontario, Canada
* Corresponding author.
E-mail address: pbeaule@ottawahospital.on.ca (P.E. Beaulé).

Orthop Clin N Am 40 (2009) 357–363
doi:10.1016/j.ocl.2009.02.002

Table 1
Baseline factors

	Age[a] (yr)	Ratio of Males to Females	Body Mass Index[a]	Preoperative Diagnosis: Osteoarthritis
HHR HRA	48.6 (29–62)	44:6	27.0 (19–40)	44/50
TSO	47.2 (30–66)	41:9	27.7 (21.5–36)	41/50
P value	0.353	0.122	0.372	0.143

[a] The values are given as the mean, with the range in parentheses.

series for both surgical approaches. No patients were excluded from this study and none lost to follow-up. No HHR patients required conversion to a more extensile approach. All patients in both the HHR and SDA group had implantation of the same hybrid resurfacing components (Conserve Plus, Wright Medical). Informed consent was obtained from all patients with approval from the institution's ethics committee.

Medical records were available for all patients and reviewed by an independent observer. Radiographs were reviewed by a blinded independent investigator who was not involved in the surgery or the aftercare of patients. The radiographic parameters recorded were the cup abduction angle, stem-to-shaft angle of the femoral component, and femoral component position in the sagittal plane.[14] All measurements were made from radiographs made at postoperative day 2.

Surgical Dislocation Approach of Ganz

The SDA, as described by Ganz and colleagues,[13] was performed on a regular operating table in the lateral position. This technique has been described in detail in a previous article.[15] In summary, a trochanteric slide osteotomy is done making sure to stay extracapsular with the osteotomy and maintaining an appropriate thickness of trochanteric slide of at least 1 cm. The slide is then mobilized anteriorly bringing the leg in flexion and external rotation exposing the hip capsule. A z-shaped capsulotomy is done and the hip dislocated anteriorly. The femoral head is usually prepared first, carefully restoring the head–neck offset, then followed by the acetabulum. Once the implants are placed, the capsule is closed and osteotomy fixed with two 4.5 mm screws. Patients are instructed to be toe-touch weight bearing for 6 weeks postoperatively to protect the trochanteric osteotomy.

Hueter-Approach Hip Resurfacing

To learn the HHR approach the senior author (P. Beaulé) visited an expert surgeon in France who then came to our institution for 1 week to assist the senior author with his first six cases, which were excluded from the present study. All cases for the HHR approach were done using an orthopedic traction table (Maquet-Dynamed, **Fig. 1**) to facilitate leg positioning for femoral head preparation and component placement. The incision is placed 1 to 2 cm postero-lateral and 2 cm distal to the anterior superior iliac spine (**Fig. 2**). The incision is extended distally and

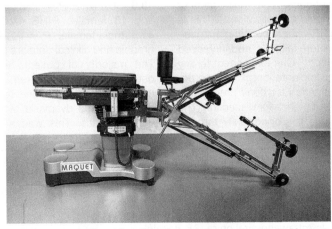

Fig. 1. Maquet-Dynamed orthopedic table with Delacroix anterior approach attachment. (*Courtesy of* Maquet-Dynamed, Inc., Markham, Ontario; with permission.)

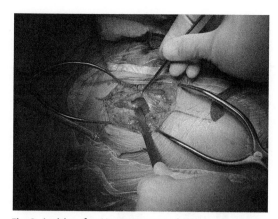

Fig. 2. Incision for Hueter approach is placed parallel and 2 cm lateral to a line extending from anterior superior iliac spine to head of the fibula. The initial dissection is done within the fascial sheath of tensor with the muscle retracted laterally.

placed postero-laterally to a line connecting to the fibular head for a total of 6 to 10 cm. The deep dissection does not differ from that described for a primary total hip replacement. However, the authors recommend releasing the reflected of rectus femoris to facilitate acetabular exposure. The lateral third of the capsule is excised. A Weber spoon is placed into the hip joint and levered on the anterior acetabular rim to dislocate the femoral head anteriorly. After a medial capsular release, the femoral head is prepared first with the leg in extension and external rotation of 180°. Final femoral component size is checked with a head spherometer gauge (**Fig. 3**). For acetabular preparation, the leg is placed in slight flexion, left to fall in external rotation, and pushed posteriorly. The use of offset reamer handles is critical for acetabular

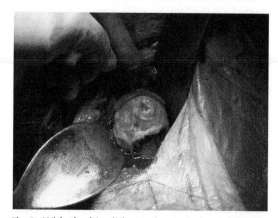

Fig. 3. With the hip dislocated anteriorly and the leg in extension and external rotation. Final sizing of the femoral head is done with the spherometer gauges (Wright Medical Technology, Memphis TN).

preparation. Before closure, an intraoperative an anteroposterior pelvis radiograph is taken (**Fig. 4**). Patients are instructed to limit weight bearing at 50% with crutches for 4 weeks. In bilateral cases, we ask the patients to walk with the aid of a walker for the same period.

The same preoperative and postoperative antibiotic therapy, thromboprophylaxis, and postoperative pain management were done in both groups (**Figs. 5** and **6**). Each patient had an intraoperative anteroposterior pelvic radiograph to confirm proper implant positioning.

Statistical Analysis

After the initial data verification, independent t-tests were used to determine differences between mean performance measures. All analyses were conducted with use of SPSS 15.0 for windows (SPSS, Chicago, Illinois). The level of significance was set at $P<.05$.

RESULTS
Operative Time

The mean operative time was longer in the SDA group than in the HHR group (109 minutes versus 93 minutes, $P<.01$). Moreover, operative time demonstrated a significant learning curve effect in the HHR group (97 minutes for the first 25 cases versus 89 minutes for the last 25 patients, $P<.01$). Comparing the first 25 HHR patients with the 50 trochanteric slide osteotomy patients, the difference was still significantly shorter (97 minutes versus 109 minutes, $P<.01$). Mean length of hospital stay ($P>.05$) and percentage of patients discharged home versus inpatient rehabilitation ($P>.05$) were not significantly different between the SDA and HHR groups: 3 and 2.98 days, respectively for length of hospital stay and 94% versus 92% for home discharges.

Radiographic Data

A significant difference was found in cup abduction angle between the two groups (**Fig. 7**). A significantly higher number of cups were positioned in the 45° to 55° range in the HHR group compared with the TSO group (19 versus 8, $P = .013$) with no cups exceeding an abduction angle of 55° in either group. The nineteen acetabular components placed at a higher abduction angle using the Hueter approach were evenly spread (10 in the first 25, 9 in the second half, $P>.05$). In five cases of the HHR, the acetabular component was repositioned to correct excessive abduction.

No significant difference was identified in the femoral components positioning in the coronal

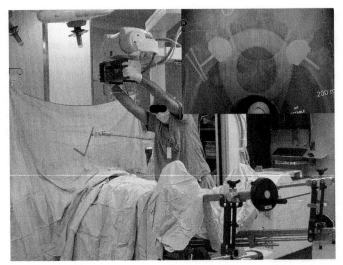

Fig. 4. Intraoperative anteroposterior radiograph is taken to confirm implant position. Inset shows quality of image.

plane (see **Fig. 1**). On the sagittal plane, a significantly higher number of components were anteriorly translated in the HHR group compared with the SDA group (14 versus 1, P<.001). A significantly higher number of components were posteriorly translated in the trochanteric slide group (19 versus 6, P<.001). There were no outliers regarding femoral component positioning, no component being in a varus position of less than 127° (**Figs. 8** and **9**).

Complications

In the SDA group, seven patients required screw removal because of trochanteric pain. Other complications in the SDA group were greater trochanter fracture requiring refixation, component mismatch, partial peroneal nerve palsy, one deep vein thrombosis, and one superficial infection requiring debridement. In the HHR group, one patient was reoperated for a retained drain

and one had deep infection requiring revision surgery. There were no deep vein thrombosis in this group. There were femoral neck fractures for the entire study group.

DISCUSSION

HRA has had resurgence in interest over the last decade as a solution for the young adult with hip arthritis maintaining femoral bone stock and permitting high levels of activity.[1,16] Because of the retained femoral head and neck, extensile approaches have been favored to optimize implant positioning and make the procedure more germane for surgeons.[17,18] The necessity of an extensile approach leaves hip resurfacing at a crossroad in regard to minimizing soft tissue trauma and time to recovery after total hip arthroplasty.[2] Of the less invasive surgical approaches

Fig. 5. Preoperative radiographs of a male 56 years of age with bilateral hip osteoarthritis. Inset shows cross table lateral of both hips.

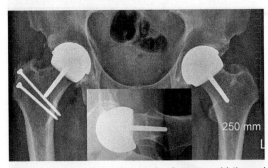

Fig. 6. Postoperative radiograph after staged bilateral hip resurfacing. The right hip was done through a surgical dislocation approach prior to starting the anterior-Hueter approach. The left hip was done one year ago through the anterior approach.

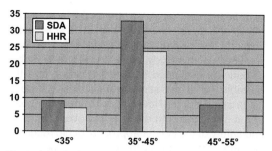

Fig. 7. Acetabular component position comparing the two approaches.

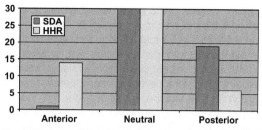

Fig. 9. Position of the femoral components in the axial plane between the two surgical groups expressed in number of hips.

to the hip, the Hueter approach is the only truly internervous approach to the hip and has a well established track record in the total hip arthroplasty literature in regard to its safety and efficacy.[11,19,20] More importantly, because the obturator externus tendon is left intact when the hip is dislocated anteriorly, the main blood supply to the femoral head (ascending branch of the medical circumflex) is not compromised.[21] Consequently, the Hueter approach cannot only fulfill the goals of soft tissue preservation but also minimizes the biologic insult to the femoral head following hip resurfacing. However, as with any new surgical technique, it is critical that the perceived advantages do not introduce unforeseen complications. The authors' initial experience with the Hueter approach did not demonstrate an increased risk of complications with comparable implant positioning and patient recovery versus the SDA. In this study, the surgical times were significantly shorter in the HHR group because of the need for reduction and fixation of the trochanteric fragment in the SDA. However, because the Hueter approach does not involve a large soft tissue dissection, closure is simple with only the fascia over tensor as a required deep layer closure. Consequently, it probably has an overall shorter surgical time. More important, once dislocated, the femoral head and neck point directly anteriorly so that the direct visualization of the femoral neck axis facilitate guide wire placement. Even though the posterior aspect of

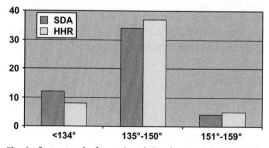

Fig. 8. Stem-to-shaft angle of the femoral component between the two surgical groups expressed in number of hips.

the femoral head and neck junction is not fully visualized and the superior neck only partially, there was no significant difference in femoral component placement in the coronal plane between the two surgical approaches. The only significant difference was a higher percentage of implants being translated anteriorly in the Hueter approach group, which is likely secondary to difficulty in clearing the iliac crest when placing the guide wire for femoral component preparation. This is advantageous in terms of minimizing the risk of postoperative hip impingement.[22] Finally, because our preference is to reference from the inferomedial neck for guide wire placement, the femoral component is automatically translated superiorly, in effect avoiding neck notching during head preparation even though the superior aspect of the femoral neck is not completely visualized with the Hueter approach.

On the other hand, acetabular component position with the Hueter had a higher percentage of components being placed in a 45° to 55° position (19/50 versus 8/50) although none of the components exceeded 55° (see **Fig. 1**). This is probably due to tethering of the cup impactor at the inferior end of the incision, which can be addressed by using a curved impactor or extending the incision distally. This is particularly important since it is becoming increasingly recognized that initial fixation and placement of the acetabular component are causes of early failure of metal-on-metal hip resurfacing. In a recent paper, Kim and colleagues[23] reported a 7.0% failure rate (14 out of 200 hips) at a meantime follow-up of 31 months with 71% (10 out of 14) of the failures occurring on the acetabular side. Most of the failures occurred with surgeons with the least amount of experience with hip resurfacing. This is probably related to the inability to insert supplement screw fixation and the difficulties in fully seating the acetabular component to obtain sufficient bony contact for ingrowth. In addition, recent reports have shown that cups placed at abduction angles of greater than 55° are associated with increased risk of higher levels of metal ion release.[9] Although what constitutes the maximum abduction cup that can be tolerated will most likely vary depending in implant design, surgeons should aim for an angle of 40° to 45°. In that respect, the relative ease of obtaining an intraoperative anteroposterior radiograph in the supine position with the Hueter approach certainly provides an additional safeguard in minimizing the risks associated with the introduction of a new surgical technique.

Although the authors' initial results with the Hueter approach are comparable to the more extensile SDA approach, what truly represents the learning curve in surgery remains to be defined. In the current surgical age of accountability, defining the learning curve of new surgical procedure is somewhat in vogue. It is based on the notion that if one had the means, there would be quantitative measure of skill that, if displayed on a chart, would show a continuous and elegant geometric curve defining the learning process.[24] In the surgical literature the learning curve is most frequently defined as a statistically significant improvement in operative time or decrease in complication rate with procedure volume. While it may seem surprising that no significant learning curve was observed, the authors relate this to a number of factors. First, the senior author is very experienced in HRA. Therefore, even through this is an unfamiliar approach, there is less new information to challenge this surgeon relative to a surgeon with less experience.[25] As a result, the functional task difficulty (challenge of the task relative to the skill level of the of the individual performing the task) is acceptable and the surgeon is likely positioned on a less steep portion of the learning curve.[25] This has several implications, first and foremost the surgeon is not likely to be overwhelmed by the task, providing a measure of safety for the patients. However, it also means that there is less information available for the expert to learn from and the slope of the learning curve is less, and perhaps less apparent over the course of 50 cases. In addition, although this was a consecutive series, the senior author used caution in introducing a new approach by being mentored for his first six cases and using intraoperative radiography to avoid gross component malposition.

In the present study, no differences between approaches were seen in the clinical parameters evaluated such as length of hospitalization and need for inpatient rehabilitation. This reflects the nonselection bias for both approaches and the relatively young age of the study group. At present, the Hueter approach is the authors' surgical approach of choice for hip resurfacing since our overall experience with the SDA of Ganz for hip resurfacing was associated with 8.7% nonunion rate of the great trochanter and an 18% reoperation rate for painful internal fixation.[26] The main weakness of this study relates to the small number of patients evaluated in the HHR group and the possibility that the senior author may still be in his learning curve. However, with the main goals of the study being to evaluate the overall efficacy and safety of the Hueter approach for hip resurfacing, the data supports the continued use of this approach with further research focusing on defining specific clinical benefits of this approach compared with the more common posterior approach.

While a learning curve likely exists for every procedure, it is more than likely surgeon dependant and based on previous operative and learning experiences. It is however, our duty as a profession to minimize its gradient. Therefore, perhaps the greatest value in defining the learning curve of specific procedures is in determining which procedures may be safely and broadly used by appropriately trained physicians. The results of this study suggest that with the experienced surgeon, with appropriate safeguards, the Hueter approach can be safely introduced without concern of significant patient complication, even if associated with a relatively complex surgical procedure such as hip resurfacing. In the introduction of new procedures, the authors strongly suggest that observation of an expert, and the use of a surgical proctor and adjunct sources of information (such as intraoperative imaging) to minimize patient risk. More importantly, we need to better standardize our definition of a learning curve to provide appropriate guidelines in order to avoid complications associated with other minimally invasive techniques.

SUMMARY

In conclusion, before commencing HRA, surgeons must be aware that there is a learning curve associated with this procedure, and are strongly urged to undertake additional training, including didactic courses, supervised cadaver dissection, independent cadaver dissection, and visits to watch surgeons who have experience with the performance of hip resurfacing operations.[1,27]

REFERENCES

1. Shimmin AJ, Beaule PE, Campbell PA. Current concepts: metal on metal hip resurfacing. J Bone Joint Surg Am 2008;90(3):637–54.
2. Ward SR, Jones RE, Long WT, et al. Functional recovery of muscles after minimally invasive total hip arthroplasty. Instr Course Lect 2008;57(57):249–54.

3. Pagnano MW, Trousdale RT, Meneghini RN, et al. Patients preferred a mini-posterior THA to a contralateral two-incision THA. Clin Orthop Relat Res 2006;453(453):156–9.

4. Meneghini RN, Pagnano MW, Trousdale RT, et al. Muscle damage during MIS total hip arthroplasty: Smith-Petersen versus posterior approach. Clin Orthop Relat Res 2006;453(453):293–8.

5. Nakata K, Nishikawa M, Yamamoto K, et al. A clinical comparative study of the direct anterior with mini-posterior approach. J Arthroplasty, in press.

6. Fehring TK, Mason JA. Catastrophic complications of minimally invasive hip surgery. A series of three cases. J Bone Joint Surg 2005;87A(4):711–4.

7. Beaule PE, Lee J, LeDuff M, et al. Orientation of femoral component in surface arthroplasty of the hip: a biomechanical and clinical analysis. J Bone Joint Surg 2004;86A(9):2015–21.

8. Shimmin A, Back D. Femoral neck fractures following Birmingham hip resurfacing. A national review of 50 cases. J Bone Joint Surg 2005;87B(3):463–4.

9. De Haan R, Pattyn C, Gill HS, et al. Correlation between inclination of the acetabular component and metal ion levels in metal-on-metal hip resurfacing replacement. J Bone Joint Surg 2008;90B(10):1291–7.

10. Pandit HP, Glyn-Jones S, McLardy-Smith P, et al. Pseudotumors associated with metal-on-metal hip resurfacings. J Bone Joint Surg 2008;90B(7):847–51.

11. Siguier T, Siguier M, Brumpt B. Mini-incision anterior approach does not increase dislocation rate: a study of 1037 total hip replacements. Clin Orthop Relat Res 2004;426(426):164–73.

12. Beaule PE, Campbell PA, Lu Z, et al. Vascularity of the arthritic femoral head and hip resurfacing. J Bone Joint Surg 2006;88A(Suppl 4):85–96.

13. Ganz R, Gill TJ, Gautier E, et al. Surgical dislocation of the adult hip. A new technique with full access to the femoral head and acetabulum without the risk of avascular necrosis. J Bone Joint Surg 2001;83B(8):1119–24.

14. Beaule PE, Dorey FJ, LeDuff MJ, et al. Risk factors affecting outcome of metal on metal surface arthroplasty of the hip. Clin Orthop 2004;418(418):87–93.

15. Beaule PE. A soft tissue sparing approach to surface arthroplasty of the hip. Operat Tech Orthop 2004;14(4):16–8.

16. Beaule PE, Antoniades J. Patient selection and surgical technique for surface arthroplasty of the hip. Orthop Clin North Am 2005;36(2):177–85.

17. Hing CB, Back D, Shimmin A. Hip resurfacing: indications, results and conclusions. Instr Course Lect 2007;56:171–8.

18. Amstutz HC, Beaule PE, Dorey FJ, et al. Metal-on-metal hybrid surface arthroplasty. Surgical Technique. J Bone Joint Surg 2006;88A(Suppl 1):234–9.

19. Matta JM, Shahrdar C, Ferguson T. Single-incision anterior approach for total hip arthroplasty on an orthopaedic table. Clin Orthop Relat Res 2004;441(441):115–24.

20. Saliari E, Leonard P, Mamoudy P. Dislocation after total hip arthroplasty using Hueter anterior approach. J Arthroplasty 2008;23(2):266–72.

21. Gautier E, Ganz K, Krugel N, et al. Anatomy of the medial circumflex artery and its surgical implications. J Bone Joint Surg 2000;82B(5):679–83.

22. Kennedy JG, Rogers WB, Soffe KE, et al. Effect of acetabular component orientation on recurrent dislocation, pelvic osteolysis, polyethylene wear, and component migration. J Arthroplasty 1998;13(5):530–4.

23. Kim PR, Beaule PE, Laflamme GY, et al. Causes of early failure in a multicenter clinical trial of hip resurfacing. J Arthroplasty 2008;23(6 Suppl 1):44–9.

24. Gallivan S. Report to the Bristol royal infirmary inquiry learning curves in relation to surgery. A Discussion Paper 2000.

25. Guadagnoli MA, Lee TD. Challenge point: a framework for conceptualizing the effects of various practice conditions in motor learning. J Mot Behav 2004;36(2):212–24.

26. Beaule PE, Shim P, Banga K. Clinical experience with the Ganz surgical dislocation approach for hip resurfacing. Dallas (TX): American Association of Hip and Knee Surgeons; 2008.

27. Marker DR, Seyler TM, Jinnah RH, et al. Femoral neck fractures after metal-on-metal total hip resurfacing: a prospective cohort study. J Arthroplasty 2007;22(7 Suppl 3):66–71.

Comparison of Mini-Incision Total Hip Arthroplasty Through an Anterior Approach and a Posterior Approach Using Navigation

Nobuhiko Sugano, MD[a],*, Masaki Takao, MD[a], Takashi Sakai, MD[a], Takashi Nishii, MD[a], Hidenobu Miki, MD[b], Nobuo Nakamura, MD[c]

KEYWORDS
- Total hip arthroplasty • Navigation
- Minimally invasive surgery
- Computer-aided surgery • Range of motion

Proponents of minimally invasive surgery (MIS) techniques for total hip arthroplasty (THA) believe that these techniques hold the promise of decreased tissue damage, blood loss, and postoperative pain; faster postoperative recovery; shortened length of stay; and improved cosmetic results.[1–3] The use of a small incision does not necessarily mean that a technique is minimally invasive; however, various currently used MIS approaches, including the two-incision approach, mini-posterior approach, mini-anterolateral approach, and mini-anterior approach all use a small skin incision. Therefore, skeptics of MIS worry about the addition of new risks to an already successful surgery; for example, poor visualization increases difficulty in prosthetic positioning and reduces the ability to thoroughly assess stability. These difficulties may result in component malpositioning, prosthetic joint instability, or increased risk of dislocation.[4]

It is always a challenge to avoid misalignment of implants in MIS. Although some MIS approaches use fluoroscopic images to guide reamers and implant inserters, fluoroscopic images are still two-dimensional guidance systems and their accuracy in measuring implant orientation is limited. To eliminate malpositioning of acetabular cups in MIS-THAs, computer navigation has been reported to be useful.[5–7] However, a question arises: as long as the cup can be oriented accurately using navigation, are there any differences among the several MIS approaches? The authors were the first to utilize navigation techniques in THA, using a mini-incision posterior approach (MPA) and a mini-incision anterior approach (MAA) on a lateral position.[8] This article reports on differences in the direction of cup insertion against the operating table, intraoperative hip range of motion (ROM), joint stability, and a choice of elevated-rim acetabular liners between an MPA and an MAA when using a CT-based navigation system.

METHODS

The authors reviewed the results of MIS-THAs performed by a single surgeon between January 2005

[a] Department of Orthopedic Surgery, Osaka University Graduate School of Medicine, Suita, Osaka 565-0871, Japan
[b] Department of Orthopedic Surgery, National Hospital Organization Osaka National Hospital, Osaka 540-0006, Japan
[c] Center of Arthroplasty, Kyowakai Hospital, Osaka 541-0001, Japan
* Corresponding author.
E-mail address: sugano@ort.med.osaka-u.ac.jp (N. Sugano).

Orthop Clin N Am 40 (2009) 365–370
doi:10.1016/j.ocl.2009.04.003
0030-5898/09/$ – see front matter © 2009 Elsevier Inc. All rights reserved.

and April 2007 using a CT-based navigation system (CT-HIP, version 1.0, Stryker Navigation, Freiburg, Germany) with the same aiming orientation for the cups. The MPA group consisted of 39 consecutive patients and the MAA group consisted of 33 consecutive patients. The skin incision ranged from 8 cm to 10 cm, with an average of 9 cm in either group. In the MPA group, repair of the external rotators was performed. In the MAA group, the Smith-Petersen interval was used.[9] The patient demographics are shown in **Table 1**. There were no significant differences in age, sex, diagnosis, height, weight, and body mass index between the two groups. In these case series, a cementless THA system was used, consisting of an anatomic, short, metaphysis-filling stem with a grit-blast hydroxyapatite coating on the proximal third of its surface, titanium-plasma-spray HA-coated cups, and Crossfire polyethylene liners (CentPillar GB and Trident, Stryker Orthopaedics, Mahwah, New Jersey). Although Trident cups with cluster holes were used, the authors used a press-fit technique without screws. The diameter of the femoral head was 32 mm.

Preoperative CT images of each patient were taken using a helical CT scanner (HiSpeed Advantage, GE Medical Systems, Milwaukee, Wisconsin) from the level of the superior anterior iliac spine of the pelvis to the level of the femoral condyles. The slice thickness was 1 mm, and the pitch was 3 mm. The CT data were transferred to the preoperative planning module of the navigation system. On the three orthogonal multiplanar reconstruction views, several landmarks of the pelvis and bone were used to segment the pelvis and femora and to define the coordinates of each bone. The pelvic coordinates were defined as follows: (1) the axial reference was referred to the anterior pelvic plane through the superior anterior iliac spines and the pubic tubercles, (2) a line through the bottom of the bilateral ischia was used to adjust the horizontal axis, and (3) the anterior-posterior axis

was tilted according to the tilt of the anterior pelvic plane when the patient was lying in a supine position on the CT table. The femoral coordinates were defined as follows: (1) the vertical axis was referred to a line through the trochanteric fossa and the knee center, and (2) the coronal plane was parallel to the table plane through the posterior prominent of the greater trochanter and the posterior femoral condyles.

For each patient, a three-dimensional surface model of the pelvis was constructed using a segmentation procedure in the planning module for intraoperative surface registration. Position and orientation of the cup was planned using three multiplanar reconstruction views and a three-dimensional volume-rendering view (**Fig. 1**). The target orientation of the cup was planned to be 40° degrees of inclination and 15° degrees of anteversion in the radiographic definition[10] because the planned stem anteversion was 30° degrees, plus or minus 10° degrees, in that series.[11]

The THA procedures were performed with the patients in a lateral position under general anesthesia. The dynamic reference markers were fixed to the pelvis using two apex pins of 3 mm in diameter and an external fixator system for the pelvis and to the lateral thigh using two percutaneous Kirschner wires of 2.4 mm in diameter and the external fixator system for the femur.

First, registration of the femur was performed. Next, after femoral head resection and acetabular exposure, registration of the pelvis was performed. Initially, coarse paired-point registration was performed by digitizing four bony landmarks, which had been determined at preoperative planning. Then, precise surface registration was performed by digitizing 30 points on the bone surface.[8] Digitizing for surface registration is performed through a skin incision using a digitizing pointer with optical sensors. After the registration process was completed, verification was determined by touching the bony surface. The position

Table 1		
Patient demographics		
	Surgical Approach (Patients)	
Patient Characteristics	**MPA Group (n = 39)**	**MAA Group (n = 33)**
Age (average ± SD)	57 ± 12	56 ± 13
Sex (female/male)	36/3	29/4
Diagnosis (osteoarthritis/osteonecrosis)	30/9	23/10
Height (cm) (average ± SD)	155 ± 6	155 ± 8
Weight (kg) (average ± SD)	55 ± 10	55 ± 11
Body mass index (average ± SD)	23 ± 4	23 ± 4

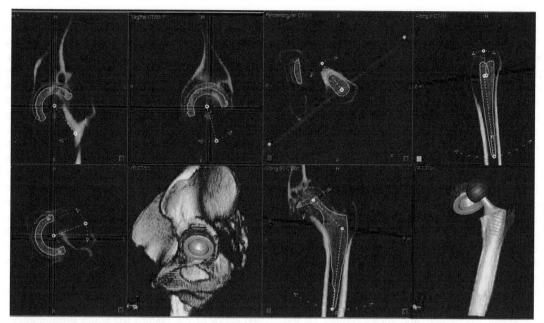

Fig. 1. Preoperative planning module using CT-Hip navigation.

of the surgical tools and the target orientation of the cup to the pelvis were verified on the monitor, and the cup was fixed using a 1.8-mm press-fit at the rim without screws. After a secure press-fit was obtained, the cup orientation was recorded using the navigation system, and the flexion angle of the cup inserter was recorded in comparison with the operating table using a goniometer.

After placement of all components, ROM and joint stability were measured using the navigation system. The maximum flexion, extension, abduction, internal rotation at 90° of hip flexion, and external rotation at 0° of extension were recorded. Joint stability was checked using the navigation system. When hip subluxation of more than 3 mm was detected during the ROM test, the navigation system changed the color of the implants on the monitor. A shuck test was performed by applying axial traction to the lower limb distally in a neutral position of the hip, and the maximum separation between the cup and the femoral head was recorded using the navigation system.

Radiographic evaluation was performed immediately after surgery, at 3 months, at 6 months,

Table 2
Intraoperative ROM and separation by traction

Intraoperative Evaluation	Surgical Approach (Patients)	
	MPA Group (n = 39)	MAA Group (n = 33)
ROM (degrees)		
Flexion (average/maximum/minimum)	98/120/62	100/122/60
Extension (average/maximum/minimum)	17/42/1	21/46/−2
Abduction (average/maximum/minimum)	32/45/14	35/45/11
Internal rotation (average/maximum/minimum)[a]	48/60/24	41/59/10
External rotation (average/maximum/minimum)[b]	16/44/−11	25/44/10
Shuck test (mm)		
Separation (average/maximum/minimum)	7/16/0	9/19/0

[a] $P<0.05$.
[b] $P<0.05$.

and annually using standardized anteroposterior and lateral radiographs of the pelvis and femur. To measure the cup orientation, an ellipse was fitted to the acetabular component rim on the early postoperative anteroposterior radiographs using computer software (CAM of THA, Kyocera, Japan).[12] To eliminate measurement error caused by pelvic axial rotation on the anteroposterior radiographs, only radiographs on which the pubic symphysis and the spinous processes of the sacrum were on a vertical line were selected for measurements. When the anteversion was less than 10°, postoperative CT images were used to judge the direction of version. The modes of determining femoral component fixation at 2 years postoperatively were classified as bone-ingrowth fixation, stable fibrous fixation, and unstable fixation, according to Engh and colleagues.[13] Migration of femoral components was determined on the basis of measurement of the vertical distance from the shoulder of the stem to the midpoint of the lesser trochanter, and measurement of the varus angle of the stem formed by the stem axis and the proximal femur axis. More than 4 mm of subsidence in the vertical distance or changes of more than 2° in the varus angle were considered to indicate stem migration and loosening. Loosening of acetabular components was defined as more than 2 mm of migration or changes of more than 5° in the abduction angle of the acetabular component.[14]

Clinical evaluation was performed preoperatively and at 6 months and 2 years postoperatively, using the Japanese Orthopedic Association hip score and the Oxford hip score.[15] The patients' rehabilitation records were also checked to identify the day when each patient was able to walk without a cane.

A χ^2 test was used for categorized data, and the Mann-Whitney U test was used for continuous data. P values of less than 0.05 were considered to be statistically significant.

RESULTS

All patients were followed for at least 2 years. There were no infections or pulmonary embolisms in either group. There were no navigation-related complications. There were no failures in using navigation, including loosening of the trackers or software or hardware errors. The average cup inclination and anteversion recorded using navigation were 38.4° (range, 33.3° to 46.6°) and 13.8° (range, 5.8° to 17.4°), respectively, in the MPA group, and 38.4° (range, 34.7° to 42.6°) and 14.8° (range, 9.4° to 22.7°), respectively, in the MAA group. There were no significant differences

in the recorded cup inclination or anteversion between the two groups. The average flexion angle of the cup inserter against the operating table was 29° (range, 22° to 38°) in the MPA group and 8° (range, −2° to 17°) in the MAA group, with a significant difference (P<0.001). Intraoperative ROM and separation by traction measurements are shown in **Table 2**. There were no significant differences between the two groups in the average flexion, extension, abduction, or separation, as determined by using a shuck test. However, the average internal rotation at 90° of flexion was significantly larger in the MPA group than in the MAA group, whereas the average external rotation was significantly smaller in the MPA group than in the MAA group. Although these differences in ROM were observed between the two groups, no instability was found. No elevated-rim acetabular liner was used in any case.

Clinically, there was no significant difference in the average Japanese Orthopedic Association hip score or the Oxford hip score preoperatively or at 6 months and 2 years of follow-up (**Table 3**). No dislocations were seen in either group. The anterior approach, however, showed a faster recovery time, which was determined by the number of postoperative days before a patient could walk 20 meters without a cane (see **Table 3**).

The average cup abduction in both groups was 40°, which was the same as the aiming angle (**Table 4**). The average cup anteversion was significantly larger in the MPA group than in the MAA group; however, the difference was less than 2°, with a relatively small standard deviation. There was no case in either group that showed cup orientation outside of the Lewinnek safe zone.[16] At 2 years of follow-up, all cases were classified as bone ingrown stable.

DISCUSSION

One of the claimed benefits of MIS is soft-tissue preservation, and the use of MIS may lead to increased stability, resulting in a reduced incidence of dislocation. On the other hand, MIS may increase a risk of implant malpositioning or malorientation, which may lead to an increased dislocation rate. In this study, the authors' wanted to identify any intraoperative or postoperative differences between the MPA and the MAA after eliminating malorientation of the cup using navigation. Although it was not always possible to acquire the target orientation of the cup even when using navigation because of undesirable effects of the press-fit procedure,[17] the authors confirmed that CT-based navigation was effective in decreasing the variation in cup orientation for

Table 3
Clinical evaluation

	Surgical Approach (Patients)	
Evaluation Criteria	MPA Group (n = 39)	MAA Group (n = 33)
Walking without a cane		
Postoperative days (average ± SD)[a]	18 ± 7	11 ± 4
Japanese Orthopedic Association hip score		
Preoperative	43 ± 15	50 ± 12
At 6 months	93 ± 6	94 ± 6
At 2 years	94 ± 5	95 ± 5
Oxford hip score		
Preoperative	34 ± 10	32 ± 10
At 6 months	17 ± 8	16 ± 5
At 2 years	16 ± 6	15 ± 4

[a] $P<0.05$.

both MPA and MAA procedures. They found two interesting differences between the two MIS approaches. First, the flexion angle of the cup inserter was significantly larger in the MPA group than in the MAA group, although the aiming cup anteversion was the same in both groups and there was little difference in the recorded cup anteversion between the two groups. The flexion angle was the same as the surgical anteversion in both groups, and a mechanical guide with 20° of surgical anteversion indicated that the surgical anteversion was 9° degrees smaller on average than the aiming angle for the MPA group and 12° larger than the aiming anteversion for the MAA group. This phenomenon can be explained by the pelvic axial rotation caused by the anterior retraction of the femur through the posterior approach for the acetabular procedure or the posterior retraction of the femur through the anterior approach.

Second, there were ROM differences in internal rotation at 90° of hip flexion and external rotation at 0° of hip flexion between the two groups. This can be explained by differences in the portion of soft-tissue release between the two groups. Because posterior soft tissues were released in the MPA group, internal rotation at 90° of hip flexion was increased, whereas external rotation was tighter in the MAA group. However, the authors did not find any differences using intraoperative joint stability tests, and they did not use an elevated-rim polyethylene liner. This means that the accurate placement of the cup using sufficient soft tissue tension may be more important for joint stability than the type of approach that is used.

When the authors compared the two approaches using navigation, they found only one benefit for using the MAA: a faster recovery when compared with the MPA in terms of the

Table 4
Postoperative cup orientation

	Surgical Approach (Patients)	
Cup Orientation	MPA Group (n = 39)	MAA Group (n = 33)
Cup inclination (degrees)		
Average ± SD	40.0 ± 2.6	40.4 ± 2.4
Maximum/minimum	49.4/35.8	44.9/35.6
Cup anteversion (degrees)[a]		
Average ± SD	13.9 ± 2.9	12.3 ± 2.8
Maximum/minimum	22.0/7.3	20.2/6.7

[a] $P<0.05$.

period until the cane was not needed for walking. However, there was no clinical benefit after 6 months.

There are some limitations in this study. First, the study was not randomized. However, the authors believe that the patients' demographic factors are unlikely to affect the results because the two groups were comparable in terms of age, gender, body mass index, and underlying disease. Second, the number of patients enrolled in this study was small, and there might be some type II errors. However, the authors believe that the two differences that they found were reliable and can provide useful information regarding either approach.

In conclusion, the mini-incision anterior approach showed a faster recovery time, but there were no differences in the incidence of dislocation or hip scores after 6 months. The intraoperative joint stability measurements showed no large difference between the two groups when malpositioning of the cup was eliminated by using navigation.

REFERENCES

1. Berger RA. Total hip arthroplasty using the minimally invasive two-incision approach. Clin Orthop Relat Res 2003;417:232–41.
2. Matta JM, Shahrdar C, Ferguson T. Single-incision anterior approach for total hip arthroplasty on an orthopaedic table. Clin Orthop Relat Res 2005;441: 115–24.
3. Wright JM, Crockett HC, Delgado S, et al. Mini-incision for total hip arthroplasty: a prospective, controlled investigation with 5-year follow-up evaluation. J Arthroplasty 2004;19(5):538–45.
4. Woolson ST, Mow CS, Syquia JF, et al. Comparison of primary total hip replacements performed with a standard incision or a mini-incision. J Bone Joint Surg Am 2004;86(7):1353–8.
5. DiGioia AM, Plakseychuk AY, Levison TJ, et al. Mini-incision technique for total hip arthroplasty with navigation. J Arthroplasty 2003;18(2):123–8.
6. Inaba Y, Dorr LD, Wan Z, et al. Operative and patient care techniques for posterior mini-incision total hip arthroplasty. Clin Orthop Relat Res 2005;441: 104–14.
7. Nogler M, Mayr E, Krismer M, et al. Reduced variability in cup positioning: the direct anterior surgical approach using navigation. Acta Orthop 2008;79(6): 789–93.
8. Hananouchi T, Takao M, Nishii T, et al. Comparison of navigation accuracy in THA between the mini-anterior and -posterior approaches. Int J Med Robot 2009;5(1):20–5.
9. Light TR, Keggi KJ. Anterior approach to hip arthroplasty. Clin Orthop Relat Res 1980;152:255–60.
10. Murray DW. The definition and measurement of acetabular orientation. J Bone Joint Surg Br 1993; 75(2):228–32.
11. Widmer KH, Zurfluh B. Compliant positioning of total hip components for optimal range of motion. J Orthop Res 2004;22:815–21.
12. Sugano N, Nishii T, Miki H, et al. Mid-term results of cementless total hip replacement using a ceramic-on-ceramic bearing with and without computer navigation. J Bone Joint Surg Br 2007;89(4):455–60.
13. Engh CA, Glassman AH, Suthers KE. The case for porous-coated hip implants: the femoral side. Clin Orthop 1990;261:63–81.
14. Callaghan JJ, Dysart SH, Savory CG. The uncemented porous-coated anatomic total hip prosthesis: two-year results of a prospective consecutive series. J Bone Joint Surg Am 1988;70: 337–46.
15. Uesugi Y, Makimoto K, Fujita K, et al. Validity and responsiveness of the Oxford hip score in a prospective study with Japanese total hip arthroplasty patients. J Orthop Sci 2009;14(1):35–9.
16. Lewinnek GE, Lewis JL, Tarr R, et al. Dislocations after total hip-replacement arthroplasties. J Bone Joint Surg Am 1978;60:217–20.
17. DiGioia AM, Jaramaz B, Blackwell M, et al. The Otto Aufranc Award. Image guided navigation system to measure intraoperatively acetabular implant alignment. Clin Orthop Relat Res 1998;355:8–22.

Complications of the Direct Anterior Approach for Total Hip Arthroplasty

Cefin Barton, MB, BCh, MRCS(Ed), FRCS(Tr&Orth)[a],
Paul R. Kim, MD, FRCSC[b],*

KEYWORDS
- Hip • Arthroplasty • Complications • Anterior approach
- Hueter

The direct anterior approach (DAA) to the adult hip is gaining in popularity and use. It is regularly used in many centers, including the authors', for procedures such as total hip arthroplasty (THA), hemiarthroplasty, hip resurfacing, and corrective procedures for femoroacetabular impingement. Advocates of the approach claim many benefits including shorter rehabilitation times, less surgical trauma due to its muscle-splitting interval, minimal soft tissue dissection, and the small size of the incision required. Due to the supine position of the patient and the nature of the approach, however, it has its own unique set of complications. The lateral femoral cutaneous nerve (LFCN) lies close to the dissection plane. Femoral exposure and preparation is very different from more conventional approaches, and component position and the relative anatomy between socket and femur during preparation must be appreciated.

The purpose of this article is to outline the potential complications of using the DAA in THA to inform surgeons of potential pitfalls and how to avoid them. The complications are conveniently classified for ease of reference.

MATERIALS AND METHODS

The authors have collated all known complications of the surgeons using the approach at their center and have reviewed cases and the current literature on this subject. Current opinions of the authors' and others' experience on how to potentially avoid these complications are also included.

INTRAOPERATIVE COMPLICATIONS
Approach-related Complications

Lateral femoral cutaneous nerve damage
The most commonly encountered complication is an LFCN injury. The nerve lies in the interval between the sartorius and tensor fascia lata (TFL) muscles and emerges from this interval or from the substance of the sartorius. Letournel[1] introduced a modification to the classic approach in 1980, which involves approaching the deep layers from within the sheath of the TFL. It is imperative to remain within the sheath of the TFL for this approach because by doing so, the chance of an LFCN injury is greatly minimized. The LFCN runs in a separate sheath until it arborizes to supply the cutaneous area of the upper lateral thigh. This arborization usually occurs distal to the area of incision. These distal branches may be put at risk if the incision is extended distally for any reason.

Circumflex vessels
The routine exposure for THA with the DAA involves the exposure and ligation of the ascending branches of the lateral femoral circumflex vessels. These vessels lie in the interval

[a] The Ottawa Hospital-General Campus, University of Ottawa, 501 Smyth Road, CCW 1650, Ottawa, Ontario, Canada
[b] Division of Orthopedics, Adult Reconstruction Unit, The Ottawa Hospital – General Campus, University of Ottawa, 501 Smyth Road, CCW 1650, Ottawa, Ontario, Canada
* Corresponding author.
E-mail address: pkim@toh.on.ca (P.R. Kim).

Orthop Clin N Am 40 (2009) 371–375
doi:10.1016/j.ocl.2009.04.004
0030-5898/09/$ – see front matter © 2009 Elsevier Inc. All rights reserved.

between the sartorius and the TFL muscles underneath the deep fascial layer. When these vessels are not properly identified and ligated, excessive bleeding during and after the procedure can occur. These vessels are somewhat variable in location and extent. They are usually seen toward the distal end of the approach and comprise a leash of vessels that is variable in number. Routine electrocauterization usually provides adequate hemostasis of these vessels. Failure to provide adequate hemostasis can contribute to continued bleeding in the field during the procedure and to an increased risk of postoperative hematoma formation.

Muscle damage

The use of this approach is such that retraction of soft tissues is vital to gain an adequate exposure of the hip. As a result, incorrect placement of retractors or incorrect direction or overzealous retraction may cause shearing damage to the TFL, rectus femoris, or both. This can be avoided by meticulous attention to the placement of retractors and the force and direction of retraction. Specialized retractors developed for minimal-incision surgery THA can help minimize injury to the muscles. These retractors have extradepth blades and curved sides that help avoid any abrasion or shearing of muscle with retraction. Most manufacturers include these retractors as standard in their minimal-incision surgery THA instrument sets.

As part of the capsular exposure, fibers of the rectus femoris are elevated off the anterior capsule. The reflected head of the rectus femoris is also sometimes released to improve exposure. If performed carefully, minimal damage to the rectus will occur with routine exposure for DAA THA.

Femoral neurovascular bundle injury

Damage to the femoral neurovascular bundle is a potential complication of the DAA. This is true only when the proper plane of dissection is not identified at the beginning of the procedure. One possible cause is if the sartorius is mistaken for the TFL at the initial outset of the procedure. Dissection will then fall medial to the sartorius and enter the femoral triangle, with the inherent risk of damage to the contents of the triangle. The key here is the identification of the TFL, which can be identified initially by its distinct white fascial sheath that visibly thickens as it progresses laterally toward the fascia over the gluteus medius. There are usually some cutaneous perforating vessels present at the posterior edge of the TFL fascia as it transitions to the fascia over the medius. These landmarks can help to confirm the correct location of the TFL and subsequent placement of the fascial incision.

Injury to the femoral nerve can also occur through incorrect placement of retractors. When placed too deep, the femoral nerve can be inadvertently compressed, leading to a neuropraxia. It is important to keep retractors immediately intra- or extracapsular to avoid compression. Placement of a retractor over the anterior acetabulum puts the nerve at highest risk of injury if it is not carefully positioned. Again, staying immediately adjacent to bone and capsule at the midpoint of the anterior acetabulum is the best method of prevention.

Access-related Complications

Reaming and cup positioning

Cup orientation and preparation is challenging when first starting to use this procedure if the surgeon is used to performing THA with the patient in a lateral decubitus position. In some cases, only a limited view of the anterior acetabular wall can be obtained, and this makes cup placement a little more difficult, especially with regard to assessment of reaming. With the patient in the supine position, the reamers are introduced over the anterior femoral shaft. Extreme care has to be taken to not lever the reamer on the femur because doing so will direct the reamer anteriorly, with the risk of reaming away the anterior wall. Also, cup version and abduction angles are best determined relative to the native pelvis and can be easily determined by palpating both anterior superior iliac spines. Having the patient in the supine position versus the lateral decubitus position is a definite advantage in such determinations. A common error is to inadvertently insert the cup in too much anteversion. There is a tendency to hold the cup inserter too vertical, which imparts excessive anteversion to the component relative to the native pelvis. Careful attention to inserter positioning or using navigation when first learning the procedure will avoid these issues.

Femoral perforation and stem positioning

Due to the nature of the approach, it is difficult to obtain direct, straight access to the femoral canal. A "straight shot" down the canal is usually not possible. Thus, there is the potential to implant the femoral stem in varus or in an anterior-to-posterior direction. This malpositioning can be avoided by using the appropriate implant and broaching instrument handles specifically designed for a DAA approach.[2] The ideal implant is one that has a reduced lateral shoulder (**Fig. 1**), avoiding the need to ream or broach significantly into the region of the greater trochanter while still

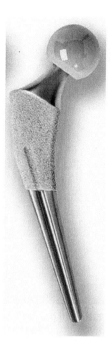

Fig. 1. Stryker Accolade stem (Stryker Orthopaedics, Mahwah, New Jersey) showing the absence of a sharp straight shoulder for ease of insertion. (*Courtesy of Stryker Orthopedics, Mahwah, NJ; with permission.*)

being able to seat the stem in a neutral position. Initial modified box chisels or "stubby" broaches (**Fig. 2**) help to gain access to the trochanteric region to avoid varus stem positioning. A more extreme complication is perforation of the femoral cortex with broaching due to malpositioning of the

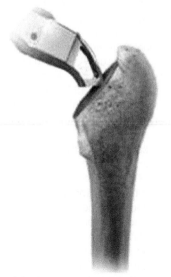

Fig. 2. A modular box osteotome (DePuy Orthopaedics) allowing controlled access to the femoral canal with minimal risk to the greater trochanter. (*Courtesy of DePuy Orthopaedics, Inc., Warsaw, IN; with permission.*)

broach. Sariali and colleagues[3] described false passages in 7 of 1374 procedures. One must be aware of how to describe these perforations, because the femur is 90° externally rotated during preparation. A posterior perforation in relation to the patient is a perforation of the lateral femoral cortex (extreme varus). This perforation occurs when the direction of the canal is not appreciated. Superior soft tissues can occasionally direct the broach in this direction. A medial perforation in relation to the patient is a perforation of the posterior femoral cortex. The anterior superior iliac spines can direct the broach handle in this direction if adequate exposure and delivery of the femur has not been fully achieved. With the use of the traction table, this exposure is enhanced by hyperextension of the hip. When the traction table is not used, it is important to perform appropriate releases to deliver the femur into the wound. The releases usually include piriformis and a partial detachment of the posterior capsule. These releases are also occasionally but less frequently required with the traction table. After the femur is delivered into the wound, a good view is obtained of the osteotomized neck to facilitate the insertion of the rasps for femoral preparation. When any concern exists, intraoperative imaging should be done to ensure proper implant or broach position (**Fig. 3**). Using a prosthesis that does not have a "straight" shoulder allows a more curved path of entry, which in turn puts less stress on the greater trochanter, thus avoiding fracture. Calcar or femoral fracture can occur with any operative approach for THA. Matta and colleagues[4] reported four proximal calcar fractures (during femoral preparation) and three greater trochanter fractures that occurred during femoral broaching or while elevating the femur with a hook. Two of the calcar fractures were successfully treated with restricted weight bearing and the other two by cerclage wiring without extending the incision. Kennon and colleagues[5] reported a total fracture rate of 2.2%, with a little over half requiring fixation. Sariali and colleagues[3] reported a fracture rate of 1.6%. Careful use of the saw to perform the initial neck cut is important. The initial neck osteotomy should be performed at an appropriate level, and one should avoid having the saw deviate into the region of the greater trochanter, which could predispose it to fracture.

Traction Table–related

Fractures

The use of a traction table for the DAA THA has been associated with injuries other than to the hip region. Matta and colleagues[4] reported

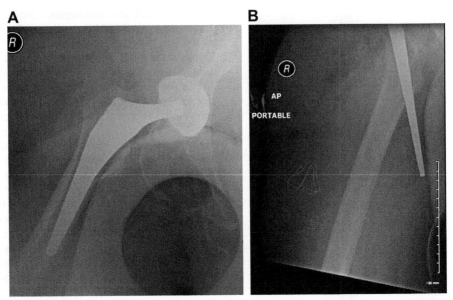

Fig. 3. (*A*) Intraoperative anteroposterior radiograph showing a problem with stem position. (*B*) Interoperative lateral radiograph confirming femoral perforation. These radiographs allowed extraction of the stem and reinsertion in the desired position, thus avoiding the need for a second procedure.

three ankle fractures with the use of the PROfx table (Orthopedic Systems Inc., Union City, California). These injuries can be avoided by not using a traction table (the senior author's preferred method) or by closely monitoring the torque applied to the ankle and tibia during dislocation and femoral preparation. The use of the traction table at the authors' unit has not led to any ankle fractures in 240 cases (Paul E. Beaulé, MD, personal communication, 2009). The fractures reported by Matta and colleagues[4] occurred during the first few months of use of the approach and the table. These investigators pointed out that minor alterations to their technique have resulted in no further fractures.

Neuropraxia

With the use of traction on any fracture table, pudendal nerve palsy is a potential complication. Although no reports of this injury with DAA THA have been published, it remains a possibility, especially with prolonged surgery and extensive traction.

POSTOPERATIVE COMPLICATIONS

Postoperative complications are mostly the same for this approach as for any other approach to the hip.

Early Postoperative Complications

Specifically, the two main early complications are dislocation and wound hematomas. Early

dislocations, as with any other approach to the hip, are usually a product of incorrect component positioning. Dislocations following the DAA are usually anterior unless the acetabular or femoral components have been significantly retroverted on implantation. Due to the musculature not being detached posteriorly or anteriorly, as long as the components are well positioned, it is postulated that inherent stability is enhanced by this approach compared with other approaches. If the precautions just stated are not heeded, however, then dislocations will inevitably occur. Reported dislocation rates by Siguier and colleagues,[6] Matta and colleagues,[4] Kennon and colleagues,[5] and Sariali and colleagues[3] were 0.96% in 1037 procedures, 0.61% in 437 hips, 1.3% in 2132 procedures, and 1.5% in 1374 procedures, respectively. These rates are significantly lower than the rates generally quoted for other approaches.

Wound hematomas and superficial wound breakdown can occur early in the postoperative period. Meticulous care should be taken with hemostasis at the end of the procedure because the only layer that is formally closed is the sheath of the TFL. Blood can therefore track from superficial to deep and vice versa when this repair is not sound. A continuous absorbable suture is used to ensure a good seal after any bleeders are coagulated. Because the wound is directly anterior, it is possible that there is less inherent pressure on the wound that may aid in hemostasis; thus, the formation of a wound hematoma in the DAA may be greater than in other approaches.

Overzealous use of retractors can damage the skin and the musculature, as mentioned earlier. The surgeon and the assistant must be constantly aware of the skin during the approach and especially during femoral preparation in THA. One must also consider body habitus in relation to the location of the incision. An obese patient who has an overhanging fat apron will have poorer skin in the proximal part of the wound to begin with, which puts their wound at risk of being under the fold or even folded over itself when the patient adopts a sitting or upright position postoperatively. This situation makes dressing the wound awkward for nursing staff. Such aspects should be taken into account when selecting patients for this approach.

Kennon and colleagues[5] reported a deep venous thrombosis rate of only 0.8% in their large series of DAA cases, a rate significantly lower than generally quoted rates. The postulated reason for this lower rate is that there is no distortion of the femoral vein during this approach compared with the posterior approach for which it is well documented that the vein is significantly distorted.

Intermediate Postoperative Complications

The only intermediate-term complication the authors have encountered is heterotopic ossification, more specifically myositis ossificans, usually within the substance of the TFL but occasionally within the rectus femoris. The authors postulate that this complication is a by-product of muscle damage secondary to retraction. The patients have not found it a problem, apart from a palpable mass in the area of the wound, and the authors have not reoperated on any of these patients. Heterotopic ossification has been seen so rarely that the authors have not deemed it necessary to use routine prophylaxis against this complication with this approach.

Finally, the authors believe that the DAA is very useful and rewarding for the patient and the surgeon. It does, however, have a significant learning curve. It is not an approach that can be easily learned from a written description and then performed well on the first attempt. It is strongly recommended that surgeons new to this approach take cadaveric training courses and have a surgeon proctor present at their first cases. Numerous courses are now available to inform surgeons of the latest advances and techniques on the DAA to THA.

REFERENCES

1. Letournel E. Acetabular fractures: classification and management. Clin Orthop Relat Res 1980;151: 81–106.
2. Nogler M, Krismer M, Hozack W, et al. A double offset broach handle for preparation of the femoral cavity in minimally invasive direct anterior total hip arthroplasty. J Arthroplasty 2006;21(8):1206–8.
3. Sariali E, Leonard P, Mamoudy P. Dislocation after total hip arthroplasty using Hueter anterior approach. J Arthroplasty 2008;23(2):266–72.
4. Matta JM, Shahrdar C, Ferguson T. Single-incision anterior approach for total hip arthroplasty on an orthopaedic table. Clin Orthop Relat Res 2004; 441(441):115–24.
5. Kennon RE, Keggi JM, Wetmore RS, et al. Total hip arthroplasty through a minimally invasive anterior surgical approach. J Bone Joint Surg Am 2003; 85(Suppl 4):39–48.
6. Siguier T, Siguier M, Brumpt B. Mini-incision anterior approach does not increase dislocation rate: a study of 1037 total hip replacements. Clin Orthop Relat Res 2004;426(426):164–73.

Multimodal Analgesia for Hip Arthroplasty

Raymond Tang, MSc, MD, FRCPC[a], Holly Evans, MD, FRCPC[b],*,
Alan Chaput, PharmD, MD, MSc, FRCPC[a], Christopher Kim, MSc[c]

KEYWORDS

- Postoperative analgesia • Hip arthroplasty
- Nonsteroidal anti-inflammatory drugs
- Cyclo-oxygenase II inhibitors • Gabapentinoids

Despite its benefits, hip arthroplasty can be associated with significant postoperative pain. Postoperative pain can adversely affect early postoperative patient recovery in several ways. Poorly controlled pain can result in sympathetic stimulation, tachycardia, or myocardial ischemia in susceptible individuals. Pain can negatively impact postoperative mobility, increasing the risk of venous thromboembolic disease. Pain also may impair rehabilitation. Any of these consequences of pain can prolong patient recovery and can increase hospital length of stay and cost. Finally, a proportion of patients who have acute postoperative pain go on to develop chronic pain conditions[1,2] that can have major negative effects on quality of life. Adequate postoperative pain management can enhance patient well-being and may minimize the physiologic consequences of pain.[3,4]

The pain experience involves a number of neurophysiologic pathways and neurochemical mediators. Multimodal analgesia represents a comprehensive approach to postoperative pain management.[5] This strategy combines analgesics with differing mechanisms of action. The goal is to target the various pathways and neurotransmitters involved in nociception. This approach may allow a reduction in the dose of each individual analgesic. For example, the use of nonopioid adjuncts can reduce opioid requirements and thereby reduce opioid-related side effects such as nausea, vomiting, sedation, respiratory depression, urinary retention, constipation, and pruritus. Furthermore, limiting intraoperative opioid use can reduce the risk of the patient's developing acute opioid tolerance.[6–8]

This article reviews the following multimodal analgesia adjuncts: acetaminophen, nonsteroidal anti-inflammatory drugs (NSAIDs), selective cyclo-oxygenase-2 (COX-2) inhibitors, gabapentinoids, tramadol, N-methyl-D-aspartate receptor antagonists, alpha-2 agonists, local anesthetic infiltration, and regional anesthesia techniques. Although a complete discussion of opioids is beyond the scope of this article, the role of neuraxial opioids is discussed. For each of the classes of analgesic adjuncts, evidence for analgesic efficacy in the hip arthroplasty population is presented when available. Recommendations for a multimodal perioperative analgesia regimen are included.

ACETAMINOPHEN

Acetaminophen is a weak analgesic that forms the most basic component of a multimodal analgesia regimen. Despite its longstanding use, the mechanism of action of acetaminophen is poorly understood. Oral administration is associated with more reliable onset (30–45 minutes) and bioavailability (79%–87%) than rectal administration.[9] The parenteral formulation is not widely available in North America. In healthy adults, hepatotoxicity can occur when more than 4 g are administered in

[a] Department of Anesthesiology, The Ottawa Hospital Civic Campus and University of Ottawa, 1053 Carling Avenue, Ottawa, Ontario, Canada. K1Y 4E9
[b] Department of Anesthesiology, The Ottawa Hospital General Campus and University of Ottawa, 501 Smyth Road, Ottawa, Ontario, Canada, K1H 8L6
[c] Division of Orthopedics, Department of Surgery, The Ottawa Hospital General Campus and University of Ottawa, 501 Smyth Road CCW 1646, Ottawa, Ontario, Canada, K1H 8L6
* Corresponding author.
E-mail address: hollyevans@sympatico.ca (H. Evans).

Orthop Clin N Am 40 (2009) 377–387
doi:10.1016/j.ocl.2009.04.001

24 hours. Dose reduction may be required in elderly patients, and its use should be limited in patients who have compromised hepatic function.

The published literature highlights the analgesic properties of acetaminophen. Two meta-analyses have investigated the effect of acetaminophen.[10,11] Studies included in these meta-analyses predominantly involved a multiple-dose regimen of parenteral acetaminophen. Approximately half of the patients included in each meta-analysis had an orthopedic surgical procedure. Acetaminophen reduced 24-hour morphine consumption by 8.3 to 9 mg compared with placebo; however, there was no difference between treatment groups in the incidence of opioid-related side effects. In a Cochrane review, Toms and colleagues[12] assessed the efficacy of a single oral dose of acetaminophen on postoperative pain based on data from 5762 patients (51 trials) undergoing various surgical procedures. They demonstrated that the number needed to treat (NNT) for a 50% reduction in visual analog pain score (VAPS) was 3.5 to 4.6 following acetaminophen, 500 to 1000 mg. These studies suggest that acetaminophen alone has a moderate impact on pain scores, a minimal impact on opioid consumption, and little effect on the incidence of opioid-related side effects.

NONSTEROIDAL ANTI-INFLAMMATORY DRUGS

The NSAIDs nonselectively inhibit the COX 1 and 2 enzymes and thereby reduce the production of inflammatory mediators such as prostaglandins and thromboxane A_2. The numerous NSAIDs available differ in onset, duration, route of administration, efficacy, and side-effect profile. Ibuprofen, for example, has nearly 100% bioavailability and reaches peak blood concentrations in 1.9 to 2.6 hours. Adverse effects of NSAIDs include platelet dysfunction, gastrointestinal mucosal damage, and renal dysfunction. Bronchospasm can occur in individuals who have asthma and nasal polyps (Sampter's triad).

Substantial evidence supports the efficacy of NSAIDs for perioperative analgesia. A meta-analysis performed by Elia and colleagues[11] included 33 trials and 2762 patients undergoing a variety of surgical procedures. Trials included various NSAID agents and dosing regimens. A single dose of an NSAID reduced 24-hour morphine consumption by 10.3 mg (95% confidence interval [CI]: −18.3 to −2.34 mg) compared with placebo. A continuous postoperative infusion of ketorolac or diclofenac had a greater impact and reduced 24-hour morphine consumption by 18.3 mg (95% CI: −26.8 to −9.74 mg). Moreover,

a multiple-dose NSAID regimen reduced 24-hour morphine consumption by 19.7 mg (95% CI: −26.3 to −13.0 mg). A multiple-dose regimen also reduced VAPS by 10 mm (95% CI: −12.5 to −7.5 mm) on a 100-mm scale. These authors found that the opioid-sparing effect of NSAIDs translated into a reduction in the incidence of nausea and vomiting from 28.8% to 22% (NNT 15; absolute risk reduction 6.8%) and a reduction in sedation from 15.4% to 12.7% (NNT 37).

The Procedure-Specific Postoperative Pain Management (PROSPECT) group[3] summarized the relevant literature on perioperative analgesia specifically for patients undergoing hip arthroplasty. They found that NSAIDs reduced morphine consumption and VAPS by 4 to 10 mm up to 32 hours postoperatively when compared with placebo.

CYCLO-OXYGENASE-2 INHIBITORS

The COX-2 inhibitors selectively inhibit the cCOX-2 enzyme and reduce production of "inducible" prostaglandins. The COX-1 enzyme is unaffected and continues to catalyze the synthesis of "homeostatic" prostaglandins. Consequently, selective COX-2 inhibitors produce analgesia and have a low incidence of associated platelet dysfunction, bleeding, and gastric ulcers.

Several systematic reviews have shown that COX-2 inhibitors improve postoperative analgesia and reduce opioid consumption in the first 24 hours.[11,13] Romsing and colleagues[14] demonstrated a 35% reduction in opioid use in their review of 19 trials that included 1606 patients having different surgical procedures. This analgesic effect was consistent across a variety of agents and dosing regimens; however, multiple doses provided the greatest benefit.[11,13–15]

Selective COX-2 inhibitors have similar benefits in the population undergoing total hip arthroplasty. Malan and colleagues[16] studied the effect of multiple doses of intravenous parecoxib, 20 or 40 mg, administered postoperatively and found that 36-hour morphine consumption was reduced by 22.1% (ie, 56.5 mg morphine) or 40.5% (ie, 43.1 mg morphine), respectively, when compared with placebo. In addition, a greater proportion of patients who received 40 mg parecoxib discontinued their opioid patient-controlled analgesia devices earlier than those receiving placebo (25.5% versus 6.2% at 24 hours, $P < .01$, and 30.9% versus 9.2% at 48 hours, $P < .01$). Similar results are evident in studies using valdecoxib, 20 to 40, mg administered twice daily,[17] rofecoxib, 50 mg, followed by 25 to 50 mg/day,[18] lumiracoxib, 400 mg, once daily,[19] and etoricoxib, 120 mg, once daily.[20]

Although both selective COX-2 inhibitors and nonselective NSAIDs are effective components of a multimodal analgesia regimen, these agents differ in their side-effect profiles and safety. In the meta-analysis by Elia and colleagues,[11] the risk of serious bleeding (defined as reoperation, blood transfusion, or severe postoperative hemorrhage) was quantified. The incidence was 0 in patients who received placebo or COX-2 inhibitors and increased to 1.7% in patients treated with NSAIDs (ketorolac, diclofenac, ketoprofen). In contrast, some COX-2 inhibitors possess adverse cardiovascular effects. The Vioxx Gastrointestinal Outcome Research (VIGOR) trial[21] compared rofecoxib, 50 mg daily, versus placebo and found that the treatment group had a fivefold higher incidence of myocardial infarction. This finding prompted the withdrawal of many COX-2 inhibitors from the market. Celecoxib and meloxicam remain in use because the cardiovascular risk associated with the use of these agents has been shown to be no higher than that associated with the use of nonselective NSAIDs. Animal research suggests that both NSAIDs and COX-2 inhibitors may reduce new bone growth by inhibiting osteoblast and osteoclast function.[22] The precise effect of small doses administered for short periods of time to humans has yet to be determined conclusively. As with any therapeutic technique, one must balance the beneficial effect with the potential for side effects.

NSAIDs and COX-2 inhibitors provide good-quality analgesia and reduce opioid requirements and opioid-related side effects. NSAIDs can be associated with a small increase in bleeding and gastritis. Both classes of drugs should be used with caution by individuals who have renal dysfunction. To obtain maximum benefit with minimal risk, it is recommended that NSAIDs and COX-2 inhibitors be used at the lowest effective dose for the shortest duration of time.

GABAPENTINOIDS

The gabapentinoid class currently includes gabapentin and pregabalin. The gabapentinoids are gamma-aminobutyric acid analogues but do not act at the gamma-aminobutyric acid receptors. They act by binding to alpha-2-delta receptors on voltage-gated calcium channels on presynaptic nerves.[23] This activity reduces the entry of calcium into presynaptic nerve terminals[24] and subsequently decreases the release of excitatory neurotransmitters such as glutamate, aspartate, substance P, and norepinephrine into the synaptic cleft. In turn, postsynaptic transmission of neural pain messages is diminished.

Most other classes of analgesics affect the transmission of neural impulses from both normal and traumatized tissues. In contrast, the gabapentinoids selectively affect the transmission of neural messages from damaged tissue.[25,26] Tissue damage leads to an increase in the number of alpha-2-delta calcium channel subunits in the dorsal root ganglia of the spinal cord.[27,28] Because the alpha-2-delta subunit is the site of action for gabapentinoids, blockade of this upregulated component of the calcium channel is postulated to be the mechanism for the enhanced effect of gabapentinoids after tissue injury.

The pharmacologic characteristics of the gabapentinoids are summarized in **Table 1**. Briefly, pregabalin offers faster onset and more reliable, dose-dependent bioavailability than gabapentin. The most common side effects of the gabapentinoids include somnolence and dizziness.[23] Headaches, balance problems, peripheral edema, and gastrointestinal symptoms also have been described. The severity of side effects following the use of pregabalin generally is dose related and can be mitigated with dose adjustment.

Gabapentinoids initially were used in the management of seizure disorders and chronic neuropathic pain. More recently, they have been used as adjuncts in the management of acute postsurgical pain in humans.[23,29] This use followed the discovery that acute postoperative pain shares some pathophysiologic features in common with chronic neuropathic pain.[23,30] For example, there is evidence that a surgical insult not only produces nociceptive pain but also leads to allodynia (a painful response to a normally nonpainful stimulus) and hyperalgesia (increased sensitivity to pain).

Several meta-analyses have documented the benefits of gabapentin in the perioperative period.[23,30–36] The meta-analysis by Tiippana and colleagues[35] included 22 studies and 1909 subjects (786 received gabapentin). The preoperative dose of oral gabapentin varied from 300 to 1200 mg. Some studies included in this meta-analysis involved the administration of a single preoperative dose of gabapentin;[37–49] in other trials, gabapentin was continued into the postoperative period.[50–57] Consequently, meta-analysis results were affected by the varied dosing regimens in the studies. Comparison of trials was complicated further because the study populations underwent varied operative procedures and therefore experienced different postoperative pain. Nevertheless, this meta-analysis concluded that gabapentin reduced opioid consumption in the first 24 hours postoperatively by 20% to 62% or by 30 ± 4 mg

Table 1
Clinical pharmacology of gabapentin and pregabalin

	Gabapentin	Pregabalin
Starting dose	100–900 mg/d	75–150 mg/d[a]
Titration	Over several weeks	Over several days
Usual effective dose	1200–2400 mg/d[a]	150–600 mg/d[a]
Maximum dose	3600 mg/d	600 mg/d
Dosage frequency	Every 8 hours	Every 8–12 hours
Time to maximal absorption	2–3 hours	0.8–1.4 hours
Oral bioavailability	42%–57%	> 90%
Metabolism	Negligible	Negligible
Elimination	Renally excreted unchanged	Renally excreted unchanged
Drug interactions	Oral antacids reduce bioavailability by 20%–30% Can potentiate other sedatives	No significant interactions Can potentiate other sedatives

[a] Reduce if patient has renal insufficiency, is elderly, there is concomitant use of other sedative medications.
    Data from Gilron I. Gabapentin and pregabalin for chronic neuropathic and early postsurgical pain: current evidence and future directions. Curr Opin Anaesthesiol 2007;20(5):456–72.

of morphine. An analysis of side effects showed that the NNT with gabapentin to prevent the opioid-related adverse effects of nausea, vomiting, and urinary retention was 25, 6, and 7, respectively. Preoperative anxiolysis was found to be a further benefit of gabapentin. In contrast, the number needed to harm for excess sedation and for dizziness was 35 and 12, respectively. The meta-analysis by Peng and colleagues[36] generated similar results. In addition, they documented that treatment with gabapentin reduced VAPS at rest (7.2–14.3 mm) and with movement (8.2–10.2 mm).

Tuncer and colleagues[46] have published the only study to date investigating the use of gabapentin for analgesia following major orthopedic surgery. These investigators randomly assigned 45 patients into one of three groups: oral gabapentin, 1200 mg, 1 hour before surgery; gabapentin, 800 mg; or placebo. All patients had standardized general anesthesia. All received intravenous patient-controlled morphine postoperatively. Pain scores and opioid consumption were evaluated at 2 and 4 hours after surgery. Both gabapentin groups had lower morphine consumption than the placebo group at 2 and 4 hours postoperatively ($P < .05$). Furthermore, the group that received 1200 mg gabapentin had reduced morphine consumption compared with the 800-mg group ($P < .05$). There was no difference in pain scores or side effects.

There has been recent interest in the perioperative use of pregabalin in the management of postoperative analgesia.[29,58–63] Mathiesen and

colleagues[61] studied 120 patients having primary hip joint replacement. All patients received spinal anesthesia with plain bupivacaine (no additives or opioids). All patients received intravenous patient-controlled analgesia with morphine in the postoperative period. Study subjects were assigned randomly to one of three groups: placebo plus placebo; pregabalin (300 mg orally) plus placebo; or pregabalin (300 mg) plus dexamethasone (8 mg intravenously). Outcomes were recorded for 24 hours following surgery. Pregabalin alone decreased 24-hour morphine consumption compared with placebo (24 ± 14 mg versus 47 ± 28 mg; $P < .003$). There was no further benefit from the addition of dexamethasone. There were no differences among groups in pain scores at rest or with movement in the first 24 hours. The addition of dexamethasone decreased the number of vomiting episodes as well as the total number of patients who vomited when compared with use of pregabalin alone ($P < .05$). Sedation scores earlier than 24 hours after surgery were higher in the pregabalin group than in the placebo group ($P < .003$), but there were no differences among groups in the incidence of dizziness.

In addition to analgesia and reduced opioid consumption, gabapentinoids may confer other ancillary benefits throughout the early perioperative period. Such advantages might include reduction in the incidence of anxiety,[40] sleep disturbance,[64] and delirium[65] as well as enhanced early postoperative joint mobility.[40] Further evidence suggests that gabapentinoids may play an important role in the prevention of chronic postoperative pain.[51,52]

OTHER ADJUNCTS

Adjuncts such as tramadol, ketamine, and clonidine may be considered for selected patients. Tramadol is a weak opioid agonist that also acts centrally by inhibiting norepinephrine and serotonin reuptake from the postsynaptic cleft. Adverse effects include nausea and vomiting, dizziness, drowsiness, sweating, and dry mouth.[66] Despite its novel mechanism of action, oral tramadol, 50 or 100 mg, did not improve VAPS, time to first analgesic request, or total analgesic use when compared with placebo in 144 patients undergoing total hip arthroplasty.[67]

Ketamine is a noncompetitive N-methyl-D-aspartate receptor antagonist. It acts centrally in the dorsal horn of the spinal cord to decrease the release of glutamate and reduce transmission of pain messages centrally. Psychotomimetic effects such as dysphoria and hallucinations can occur; however, adverse effects are less common and less severe when small doses are used.[68] Intravenous ketamine (1 mg/kg) provides analgesia, reduces 24-hour opioid requirements by 30% to 50%, and decreases the incidence of opioid-related nausea and vomiting.[68–70] Furthermore, 0.1 to 0.15 mg/kg intravenously improved early passive joint mobilization and hastened recovery in a group of patients having knee surgery.[71,72]

Clonidine is an agonist at presynaptic alpha-2 adrenoreceptors. It reduces norepinephrine release from nerve endings; as a result, pain messages are inhibited. Several studies have investigated the effect of neuraxial clonidine in patients having total hip arthroplasty. Epidural clonidine, 40 to 50 µg/hour, decreases VAPS and reduces early (24-hour) postoperative morphine requirements by up to 60%.[73,74] Although intrathecal clonidine (75 or 100 µg) can potentiate the local anesthetic's sensorimotor block, its analgesic effect is inferior to that of intrathecally administered morphine.[75] Sedation, bradycardia, and hypotension are potential side effects and may be dose limiting.[73,76]

LOCAL ANESTHETIC INFILTRATION

Local anesthetics block axonal sodium channels and inhibit the conduction of pain messages. Wound infiltration with local anesthetic acts locally to reduce peripheral nociception and is generally safe and devoid of systemic adverse effects. Local anesthetic can be placed either in the surgical incision and/or in the periarticular tissues.

Incisional Local Anesthetic

Liu and colleagues[77] undertook a meta-analysis of studies involving continuous infusion of local anesthetic into the surgical wound. They included patients having a variety of surgical procedures and found that this technique provided effective analgesia, reduced opioid requirements, and decreased the incidence of postoperative nausea and vomiting compared with placebo. A subgroup analysis of orthopedic patients (n = 458) was performed. Although the wound catheter provided no advantage when pain scores and opioid requirements were considered, the technique was associated with greater patient satisfaction and reduced hospital length of stay (weighted mean difference [95% CI] × 2.5 d [−2.8 to −2.1 d], $P <$ .001) in this subpopulation. Of the 1814 patients included in this meta-analysis, none developed local anesthetic systemic toxicity. Furthermore, there was no statistical difference between wound infection rates in the treatment and placebo groups (0.7% and 1.2%, respectively). The only study of patients undergoing total hip or knee arthroplasty patients included in this meta-analysis was the report by Bianconi and colleagues.[78] Thirty-seven patients were included in this study. The protocol involved wound infiltration with 40 mL of 0.5% ropivicaine. Subsequently, a catheter was placed between the muscle fascia and the subcutaneous tissue. Ropivicaine 0.2% was infused through the catheter at a rate of 5 mL/hour for 55 hours. Investigators found that this treatment lowered postoperative pain at rest and with mobilization, decreased opioid requirements, and reduced hospital length of stay when compared with placebo.

Periarticular Local Anesthetic

Several studies have investigated the periarticular injection of local anesthetic in patients undergoing total hip and knee arthroplasty.[79–81] Parvataneni and colleagues[79] studied 71 patients undergoing total hip arthroplasty and 60 patients undergoing total knee arthroplasty. Patients were assigned randomly to receive an intravenous opioid patient-controlled analgesia device or an intraoperative periarticular injection of 40 to 80 mL of 0.5% bupivicaine with 4 to 10 mg morphine, 40 mg methylprednisolone, 750 mg cefuroxime, and 300 mcg epinephrine. The group that received the periarticular injection of local anesthetic demonstrated improvements in analgesia and early postoperative recovery. More patients in the local anesthetic group were able to perform a straight-leg raise on the first postoperative day (52% versus 15%, $P <$ .05). Furthermore, hospital length of stay was shorter in the local anesthetic group (3.2 days versus 4.2 days, $P < .05$). In another study, Andersen and colleagues[81] compared epidural analgesia versus intra-articular injection in 80 patients having total hip arthroplasty. Patients randomly assigned to the intra-articular injection received an intraoperative dose of 151.5 mL of 0.2% ropivicaine with 30 mg ketorolac and 0.5 mg adrenaline. An indwelling intra-articular catheter was re-dosed 8 hours later with 21.5 mL of 0.7% ropivicaine, 30 mg ketorolac, and 0.5 mg adrenaline. Patients in the intra-articular injection group had lower VAPS at rest and with activity from 24 to 96 hours postoperatively and had reduced cumulative opioid consumption for 96 hours. The intra-articular group also had better-preserved lower extremity motor function as measured by Bromage score (no motor block in 100%, versus 51% of the epidural group; $P < .001$). The advantages of the intra-articular injection translated into a shorter hospital stay (4.5 days versus 7 days; $P < .001$).

Wound and periarticular local anesthetic infiltration provide site-specific analgesia with few adverse systemic effects. These techniques enhance dynamic pain management and improve postoperative mobility. Nevertheless, concerns about tissue necrosis, surgical wound infection, and chondrotoxicity[82,83] related to these techniques requires further investigation.

PERIPHERAL NERVE BLOCKS

Several authors have reported the use of a lumbar plexus block with or without sciatic nerve block for analgesia following hip arthroplasty.[84,85] Peripheral nerve blocks provide as good-quality analgesia as epidurals and are superior to systemic opioids for pain relief.[84] Peripheral nerve blocks are associated with preserved contralateral limb strength that may facilitate postoperative rehabilitation when compared with the bilateral lower extremity sensorimotor block that can result with epidural analgesia. Furthermore, hypotension and urinary retention may occur less frequently with peripheral nerve blocks than with epidurals. Peripheral nerve blocks have been used as part of a multimodal analgesia regimen to limit hospital length of stay to 23 to 48 hours following elective hip arthroplasty.[86,87] Despite these advantages, the placement of lumbar plexus and sciatic nerve blocks requires advanced regional anesthesia skills. They can have serious potential side effects including patient falls and injury,[88] nerve injury,[89] neuraxial block, systemic absorption of local anesthetic, and retroperitoneal hematoma.

NEURAXIAL ANESTHESIA

Spinal or epidural anesthesia is administered frequently for total hip arthroplasty because of advantages such as decreased intraoperative blood loss and reduced incidence of postoperative thrombotic complications.[90] Neuraxial techniques also are beneficial for postoperative analgesia. A single 0.1- to 0.2-mg dose of intrathecal morphine administered at the time of spinal anesthesia reduces VAPS and postoperative opioid consumption for 16 hours when compared with placebo.[3] Nonetheless, intrathecal opioids can be associated with typical opioid-related side effects. In the authors' practice, multimodal nonopioid analgesia in combination with low-dose intrathecal morphine can minimize such side effects.

Continuous epidural infusion of a solution of local anesthetic with or without an opioid can be used for postoperative analgesia. Choi and colleagues[91] conducted a Cochrane review comparing epidural analgesia versus parenteral opioid analgesia following lower limb arthroplasty. They observed that epidural analgesia was associated with lower VAPS in the early postoperative period and a decreased incidence of sedation. Epidural analgesia, however, was associated with a greater incidence of urinary retention, pruritus, and hypotension. Although not addressed in this meta-analysis, excessive motor block limiting postoperative mobilization represents a potential deterrent to the wider application of this technique for patients undergoing hip arthroplasty. Furthermore, epidural hematoma, which is a rare but potentially disastrous complication of epidural analgesia, remains a concern among patients having hip arthroplasty who receive postoperative thromboprophylaxis.

COMPREHENSIVE MULTIMODAL ANALGESIA REGIMEN

The Ottawa Hospital's Multimodal Analgesia Protocol is summarized in **Table 2**. The authors have found that this regimen provides excellent static and dynamic postoperative pain management with limited adverse effects.

SUMMARY

Multimodal analgesia incorporates the use of analgesic adjuncts with different mechanisms of action to enhance postoperative pain management. Adjuncts typically are administered at regular dosing intervals for several days throughout the perioperative period.

Table 2
The Ottawa Hospital multimodal analgesia protocol for hip arthroplasty

Analgesia	Regimen
Opioid-naïve patients	
Acetaminophen	650–1000 mg by mouth every 6 hours
Celecoxib	200 mg by mouth every 12 hours If sensitivity: Ibuprofen, 200–400 mg, by mouth every 4–6 hours OR Ketorolac, 15 mg, intravenously every 6 hours
Pregabalin	25–75 mg by mouth every 8 hours
Periarticular local anesthetic infiltration	Dilute solution of local anesthetic ± opioid ± ketorolac ± epinephrine
Intrathecal morphine	0.05–0.1 mg
For patients who are opioid tolerant or have chronic pain, the following agents can be added	
Tramacet	1–2 tablets by mouth every 6 hours Each tablet contains 37.5 mg tramadol + 325 mg acetaminophen Use instead of plain acetaminophen
Ketamine	0.1–0.15 mg/kg intravenous boluses as needed
Clonidine	0.1 mg by mouth daily
Lumbar plexus ± sciatic nerve block	—

Courtesy of The Ottawa Hospital General Campus, 501 Smyth Rd., Ottawa, ON, Canada K1H 8L6.

Acetaminophen is the most basic element of a multimodal analgesia regimen. This agent is a weak analgesic with minimal opioid-sparing ability but is extremely safe. In the absence of contraindications, an NSAID or COX-2 inhibitor is added. Regular dosing significantly lowers VAPS,[3] decreases opioid consumption,[3,11,13,16–20] reduces opioid-related side effects,[11] and enhances postoperative mobility. Selective COX-2 inhibitors have minimal adverse gastrointestinal and hemostatic effects; consequently, these agents may be preferred in the perioperative setting. The gabapentinoids are effective postoperative analgesics that reduce opioid consumption by up to 50% compared with placebo.[61] Pregabalin offers a more reliable dose–response relationship than gabapentin. Side effects including sedation can be minimized with dose reduction. The analgesic efficacy of tramadol in the arthroplasty population has yet to be proven. Ketamine and clonidine can be associated with significant adverse effects. Consequently, the use of these three agents generally is limited to patients who have difficult-to-manage pain, chronic pain, or opioid tolerance.

Local anesthetic-based techniques for postoperative pain management provide site-specific analgesia devoid of major systemic effects.

Periarticular local anesthetic infiltration provides more comprehensive analgesia than obtained with simple surgical wound infiltration.[77,92] Placement of a periarticular catheter enables continuous or repeated dosing that extends the duration of effect. By providing excellent dynamic pain control, this technique has been shown to have significant advantages in postoperative mobility and rehabilitation.[79,81] Nevertheless, concerns about wound infection or chondrocyte damage induced by the local anesthetic may limit more widespread use of periarticular local anesthetic infiltration.[82,83] Peripheral nerve blocks and epidural anesthesia also offer site-specific analgesia with excellent dynamic pain control. These regional anesthesia techniques have contraindications and side effects that may limit their global application. In the authors' institution, the use of peripheral nerve blocks and epidural analgesia generally is limited to patients who have difficult-to-manage pain, chronic pain, or opioid tolerance.

Opioids are the final class of analgesics that are incorporated into a multimodal regimen. Intrathecal morphine offers excellent-quality analgesia of extended duration. In combination with other adjuncts, small doses are effective and are associated with a low incidence of side effects. Oral and/or parenteral opioids are added to the multimodal analgesia regimen on an as-needed basis. The goal is to minimize opioid requirements and thereby minimize associated side effects.

The studies conducted to date are helpful when establishing an evidence-based approach to effective multimodal analgesia following hip arthroplasty. It is hoped that future investigations will involve the use of two or more analgesic adjuncts so that a truly multimodal regimen can be evaluated in terms of analgesic efficacy, dose requirements, and side-effect profile.

REFERENCES

1. Williams O, Fitzpatrick R, Hajat S, et al. Mortality, morbidity, and 1-year outcomes of primary elective total hip arthroplasty. J Arthroplasty 2002;17(2):165–71.

2. Nikolajsen L, Brandsborg B, Lucht U, et al. Chronic pain following total hip arthroplasty: a nationwide questionnaire study. Acta Anaesthesiol Scand 2006;50(4):495–500.

3. Fischer HB, Simanski CJ. A procedure-specific systematic review and consensus recommendations for analgesia after total hip replacement. Anaesthesia 2005;60(12):1189–202.

4. Buvanendran A, Kroin JS, Tuman KJ, et al. Effects of perioperative administration of a selective cyclooxygenase 2 inhibitor on pain management and recovery of function after knee replacement: a randomized controlled trial. JAMA 2003;290(18):2411–8.

5. Kehlet H, Dahl JB. The value of "multimodal" or "balanced analgesia" in postoperative pain treatment. Anesth Analg 1993;77(5):1048–56.

6. Guignard B, Bossard AE, Coste C, et al. Acute opioid tolerance: intraoperative remifentanil increases postoperative pain and morphine requirement. Anesthesiology 2000;93(2):409–17.

7. Mao J. Opioid-induced abnormal pain sensitivity: implications in clinical opioid therapy. Pain 2002;100(3):213–7.

8. Chia YY, Liu K, Wang JJ, et al. Intraoperative high dose fentanyl induces postoperative fentanyl tolerance. Can J Anaesth 1999;46(9):872–7.

9. Ameer B, Divoll M, Abernethy DR, et al. Absolute and relative bioavailability of oral acetaminophen preparations. J Pharm Sci 1983;72(8):955–8.

10. Remy C, Marret E, Bonnet F. Effects of acetaminophen on morphine side-effects and consumption after major surgery: meta-analysis of randomized controlled trials. Br J Anaesth 2005;94(4):505–13.

11. Elia N, Lysakowski C, Tramer MR. Does multimodal analgesia with acetaminophen, nonsteroidal antiinflammatory drugs, or selective cyclooxygenase-2 inhibitors and patient-controlled analgesia morphine offer advantages over morphine alone? Meta-analyses of randomized trials. Anesthesiology 2005;103(6):1296–304.

12. Toms L, McQuay HJ, Derry S, et al. Single dose oral paracetamol (acetaminophen) for postoperative pain in adults. Cochrane Database Syst Rev 2008;4:CD004602.

13. Romsing J, Moiniche S. A systematic review of COX-2 inhibitors compared with traditional NSAIDs, or different COX-2 inhibitors for post-operative pain. Acta Anaesthesiol Scand 2004;48(5):525–46.

14. Romsing J, Moiniche S, Mathiesen O, et al. Reduction of opioid-related adverse events using opioid-sparing analgesia with COX-2 inhibitors lacks documentation: a systematic review. Acta Anaesthesiol Scand 2005;49(2):133–42.

15. Straube S, Derry S, McQuay HJ, et al. Effect of preoperative Cox-II-selective NSAIDs (coxibs) on postoperative outcomes: a systematic review of randomized studies. Acta Anaesthesiol Scand 2005;49(5):601–13.

16. Malan TP Jr, Marsh G, Hakki SI, et al. Parecoxib sodium, a parenteral cyclooxygenase 2 selective inhibitor, improves morphine analgesia and is opioid-sparing following total hip arthroplasty. Anesthesiology 2003;98(4):950–6.

17. Camu F, Beecher T, Recker DP, et al. Valdecoxib, a COX-2-specific inhibitor, is an efficacious, opioid-sparing analgesic in patients undergoing hip arthroplasty. Am J Ther 2002;9(1):43–51.

18. Reicin A, Brown J, Jove M, et al. Efficacy of single-dose and multidose rofecoxib in the treatment of post-orthopedic surgery pain. Am J Orthop 2001;30(1):40–8.

19. Chan VW, Clark AJ, Davis JC, et al. The post-operative analgesic efficacy and tolerability of lumiracoxib compared with placebo and naproxen after total knee or hip arthroplasty. Acta Anaesthesiol Scand 2005;49(10):1491–500.

20. Rasmussen GL, Malmstrom K, Bourne MH, et al. Etoricoxib provides analgesic efficacy to patients after knee or hip replacement surgery: a randomized, double-blind, placebo-controlled study. Anesth Analg 2005;101(4):1104–11.

21. Bombardier C, Laine L, Reicin A, et al. Comparison of upper gastrointestinal toxicity of rofecoxib and naproxen in patients with rheumatoid arthritis. VIGOR Study Group. N Engl J Med 2000;343(21):1520–8.

22. Harder AT, An YH. The mechanisms of the inhibitory effects of nonsteroidal anti-inflammatory drugs on bone healing: a concise review. J Clin Pharmacol 2003;43(8):807–15.

23. Gilron I. Gabapentin and pregabalin for chronic neuropathic and early postsurgical pain: current evidence and future directions. Curr Opin Anaesthesiol 2007;20(5):456–72.

24. Fink K, Dooley DJ, Meder WP, et al. Inhibition of neuronal Ca(2+) influx by gabapentin and

pregabalin in the human neocortex. Neuropharmacology 2002;42(2):229–36.

25. Fehrenbacher JC, Taylor CP, Vasko MR. Pregabalin and gabapentin reduce release of substance P and CGRP from rat spinal tissues only after inflammation or activation of protein kinase C. Pain 2003; 105(1–2):133–41.

26. Li CY, Zhang XL, Matthews EA, et al. Calcium channel alpha2delta1 subunit mediates spinal hyperexcitability in pain modulation. Pain 2006; 125(1–2):20–34.

27. Luo ZD, Chaplan SR, Higuera ES, et al. Upregulation of dorsal root ganglion (alpha)2(delta) calcium channel subunit and its correlation with allodynia in spinal nerve-injured rats. J Neurosci 2001;21(6): 1868–75.

28. Newton RA, Bingham S, Case PC, et al. Dorsal root ganglion neurons show increased expression of the calcium channel alpha2delta-1 subunit following partial sciatic nerve injury. Brain Res Mol Brain Res 2001;95(1–2):1–8.

29. Hill CM, Balkenohl M, Thomas DW, et al. Pregabalin in patients with postoperative dental pain. Eur J Pain 2001;5(2):119–24.

30. Dahl JB, Mathiesen O, Moiniche S. 'Protective premedication': an option with gabapentin and related drugs? A review of gabapentin and pregabalin in in the treatment of post-operative pain. Acta Anaesthesiol Scand 2004;48(9):1130–6.

31. Ho KY, Gan TJ, Habib AS. Gabapentin and postoperative pain—a systematic review of randomized controlled trials. Pain 2006;126(1–3):91–101.

32. Hurley RW, Cohen SP, Williams KA, et al. The analgesic effects of perioperative gabapentin on postoperative pain: a meta-analysis. Reg Anesth Pain Med 2006;31(3):237–47.

33. Mathiesen O, Moiniche S, Dahl JB. Gabapentin and postoperative pain: a qualitative and quantitative systematic review, with focus on procedure. BMC Anesthesiol 2007;7:6.

34. Seib RK, Paul JE. Preoperative gabapentin for postoperative analgesia: a meta-analysis. Can J Anaesth 2006;53(5):461–9.

35. Tiippana EM, Hamunen K, Kontinen VK, et al. Do surgical patients benefit from perioperative gabapentin/pregabalin? A systematic review of efficacy and safety. Anesth Analg 2007;104(6):1545–56.

36. Peng PWH, Wijeysundera DN, Li CCF. Use of gabapentin for perioperative pain control—a meta-analysis. Pain Res Manag 2007;12(2):85–92.

37. Al-Mujadi H, A-Refai AR, Katzarov MG, et al. Preemptive gabapentin reduces postoperative pain and opioid demand following thyroid surgery. Can J Anaesth 2006;53(5):268–73.

38. Dirks J, Fredensborg BB, Christensen D, et al. A randomized study of the effects of single-dose gabapentin versus placebo on postoperative pain and morphine consumption after mastectomy. Anesthesiology 2002;97(3):560–4.

39. Rorarius MG, Mennander S, Suominen P, et al. Gabapentin for the prevention of postoperative pain after vaginal hysterectomy. Pain 2004; 110(1–2):175–81.

40. Menigaux C, Adam F, Guignard B, et al. Preoperative gabapentin decreases anxiety and improves early functional recovery from knee surgery. Anesth Analg 2005;100(5):1394–9.

41. Pandey CK, Navkar DV, Giri PJ, et al. Evaluation of the optimal preemptive dose of gabapentin for postoperative pain relief after lumbar diskectomy: a randomized, double-blind, placebo-controlled study. J Neurosurg Anesthesiol 2005;17(2):65–8.

42. Pandey CK, Priye S, Singh S, et al. Preemptive use of gabapentin significantly decreases postoperative pain and rescue analgesic requirements in laparoscopic cholecystectomy. Can J Anaesth 2004; 51(4):358–63.

43. Pandey CK, Sahay S, Gupta D, et al. Preemptive gabapentin decreases postoperative pain after lumbar discoidectomy. Can J Anaesth 2004;51(10): 986–9.

44. Pandey CK, Singhal V, Kumar M, et al. Gabapentin provides effective postoperative analgesia whether administered pre-emptively or post-incision. Can J Anaesth 2005;52(8):827–31.

45. Radhakrishnan M, Bithal PK, Chaturvedi A. Effect of preemptive gabapentin on postoperative pain relief and morphine consumption following lumbar laminectomy and discectomy: a randomized, double-blinded, placebo-controlled study. J Neurosurg Anesthesiol 2005;17(3):125–8.

46. Tuncer S, Bariskaner H, Reisli R, et al. Effect of gabapentin on postoperative pain: a randomized, placebo-controlled clinical study. Pain Clin 2005; 17(1):95–9.

47. Turan A, Karamanlioglu B, Memis D, et al. The analgesic effects of gabapentin after total abdominal hysterectomy. Anesth Analg 2004;98(5):1370–3.

48. Turan A, Karamanlioglu B, Memis D, et al. Analgesic effects of gabapentin after spinal surgery. Anesthesiology 2004;100(4):935–8.

49. Turan A, Memis D, Karamanlioglu B, et al. The analgesic effects of gabapentin in monitored anesthesia care for ear-nose-throat surgery. Anesth Analg 2004; 99(2):375–8.

50. Dierking G, Duedahl TH, Rasmussen ML, et al. Effects of gabapentin on postoperative morphine consumption and pain after abdominal hysterectomy: a randomized, double-blind trial. Acta Anaesthesiol Scand 2004;48(3):322–7.

51. Fassoulaki A, Stamatakis E, Petropoulos G, et al. Gabapentin attenuates late but not acute pain after abdominal hysterectomy. Eur J Anaesthesiol 2006; 23(2):136–41.

52. Fassoulaki A, Triga A, Melemeni A, et al. Multimodal analgesia with gabapentin and local anesthetics prevents acute and chronic pain after breast surgery for cancer [see comment]. Anesth Analg 2005; 101(5):1427–32.

53. Fassoulaki A, Patris K, Sarantopoulos C, et al. The analgesic effect of gabapentin and mexiletine after breast surgery for cancer. Anesth Analg 2002; 95(4):985–91.

54. Gilron I, Orr E, Tu D, et al. A placebo-controlled randomized clinical trial of perioperative administration of gabapentin, rofecoxib and their combination for spontaneous and movement-evoked pain after abdominal hysterectomy. Pain 2005;113(1–2):191–200.

55. Mikkelsen S, Hilsted KL, Andersen PJ, et al. The effect of gabapentin on post-operative pain following tonsillectomy in adults. Acta Anaesthesiol Scand 2006;50(7):809–15.

56. Turan A, Kaya G, Karamanlioglu B, et al. Effect of oral gabapentin on postoperative epidural analgesia. Br J Anaesth 2006;96(2):242–6.

57. Turan A, White PF, Karamanlioglu B, et al. Gabapentin: an alternative to the cyclooxygenase-2 inhibitors for perioperative pain management. Anesth Analg 2006;102(1):175–81.

58. Agarwal A, Gautam S, Gupta D, et al. Evaluation of a single preoperative dose of pregabalin for attenuation of postoperative pain after laparoscopic cholecystectomy. Br J Anaesth 2008;101(5):700–4.

59. Jokela R, Ahonen J, Tallgren M, et al. Premedication with pregabalin 75 or 150 mg with ibuprofen to control pain after day-case gynaecological laparoscopic surgery. Br J Anaesth 2008;100(6): 834–40.

60. Jokela R, Ahonen J, Tallgren M, et al. A randomized controlled trial of perioperative administration of pregabalin for pain after laparoscopic hysterectomy. Pain 2008;134(1–2):106–12.

61. Mathiesen O, Jacobsen LS, Holm HE, et al. Pregabalin and dexamethasone for postoperative pain control: a randomized controlled study in hip arthroplasty. Br J Anaesth 2008;101(4):535–41.

62. Paech MJ, Goy R, Chua S, et al. A randomized, placebo-controlled trial of preoperative oral pregabalin for postoperative pain relief after minor gynecological surgery. Anesth Analg 2007;105(5): 1449–53.

63. Mathiesen O, Rasmussen ML, Dierking G, et al. Pregabalin and dexamethasone in combination with paracetamol for postoperative pain control after abdominal hysterectomy. a randomized clinical trial. Acta Anaesthesiol Scand 2009;53:227–35.

64. Sabatowski R, Galvez R, Cherry DA, et al. Pregabalin reduces pain and improves sleep and mood disturbances in patients with post-herpetic neuralgia: results of a randomised, placebo-controlled clinical trial. Pain 2004;109(1–2):26–35.

65. Leung JM, Sands LP, Rico M, et al. Pilot clinical trial of gabapentin to decrease postoperative delirium in older patients. Neurology 2006;67(7):1251–3.

66. Scott LJ, Perry CM. Tramadol: a review of its use in perioperative pain. Drugs 2000;60(1):139–76.

67. Stubhaug A, Grimstad J, Breivik H. Lack of analgesic effect of 50 and 100 mg oral tramadol after orthopaedic surgery: a randomized, double-blind, placebo and standard active drug comparison. Pain 1995;62(1):111–8.

68. Bell RF, Dahl JB, Moore RA, et al. Perioperative ketamine for acute postoperative pain. Cochrane Database Syst Rev 2006;(1):CD004603.

69. Elia N, Tramer MR. Ketamine and postoperative pain—a quantitative systematic review of randomised trials. Pain 2005;113(1–2):61–70.

70. Kohrs R, Durieux ME. Ketamine: teaching an old drug new tricks. Anesth Analg 1998;87(5):1186–93.

71. Menigaux C, Fletcher D, Dupont X, et al. The benefits of intraoperative small-dose ketamine on postoperative pain after anterior cruciate ligament repair. Anesth Analg 2000;90(1):129–35.

72. Menigaux C, Guignard B, Fletcher D, et al. Intraoperative small-dose ketamine enhances analgesia after outpatient knee arthroscopy. Anesth Analg 2001;93(3):606–12.

73. Dobrydnjov I, Axelsson K, Gupta A, et al. Improved analgesia with clonidine when added to local anesthetic during combined spinal-epidural anesthesia for hip arthroplasty: a double-blind, randomized and placebo-controlled study. Acta Anaesthesiol Scand 2005;49(4):538–45.

74. Milligan KR, Convery PN, Weir P, et al. The efficacy and safety of epidural infusions of levobupivacaine with and without clonidine for postoperative pain relief in patients undergoing total hip replacement. Anesth Analg 2000;91(2):393–7.

75. Fogarty DJ, Carabine UA, Milligan KR. Comparison of the analgesic effects of intrathecal clonidine and intrathecal morphine after spinal anaesthesia in patients undergoing total hip replacement. Br J Anaesth 1993;71(5):661–4.

76. Grace D, Bunting H, Milligan KR, et al. Postoperative analgesia after co-administration of clonidine and morphine by the intrathecal route in patients undergoing hip replacement. Anesth Analg 1995;80(1): 86–91.

77. Liu SS, Richman JM, Thirlby RC, et al. Efficacy of continuous wound catheters delivering local anesthetic for postoperative analgesia: a quantitative and qualitative systematic review of randomized controlled trials. J Am Coll Surg 2006;203(6): 914–32.

78. Bianconi M, Ferraro L, Traina GC, et al. Pharmacokinetics and efficacy of ropivacaine continuous wound instillation after joint replacement surgery. Br J Anaesth 2003;91(6):830–5.

79. Parvataneni HK, Shah VP, Howard H, et al. Controlling pain after total hip and knee arthroplasty using a multimodal protocol with local periarticular injections: a prospective randomized study. J Arthroplasty 2007;22(6 Suppl 2):33–8.

80. Toftdahl K, Nikolajsen L, Haraldsted V, et al. Comparison of peri- and intraarticular analgesia with femoral nerve block after total knee arthroplasty: a randomized clinical trial. Acta Orthop 2007;78(2):172–9.

81. Andersen KV, Pfeiffer-Jensen M, Haraldsted V, et al. Reduced hospital stay and narcotic consumption, and improved mobilization with local and intraarticular infiltration after hip arthroplasty: a randomized clinical trial of an intraarticular technique versus epidural infusion in 80 patients. Acta Orthop 2007; 78(2):180–6.

82. Brown SL, Morrison AE. Local anesthetic infusion pump systems adverse events reported to the food and drug administration. Anesthesiology 2004;100:1305–6.

83. Gomoll AH, Kang RW, Williams JM, et al. Chondrolysis after continuous intra-articular bupivacaine infusion: an experimental model investigating chondrotoxicity in the rabbit shoulder. Arthroscopy 2006; 22(8):813–9.

84. Horlocker TT, Kopp SL, Pagnano MW, et al. Analgesia for total hip and knee arthroplasty: a multimodal pathway featuring peripheral nerve block. J Am Acad Orthop Surg 2006;14(3):126–35.

85. Buckenmaier CC 3rd, Xenos JS, Nilsen SM. Lumbar plexus block with perineural catheter and sciatic nerve block for total hip arthroplasty. J Arthroplasty 2002;17(4):499–502.

86. Hebl JR, Kopp SL, Ali MH, et al. A comprehensive anesthesia protocol that emphasizes peripheral nerve blockade for total knee and total hip arthroplasty. J Bone Joint Surg Am 2005;87(Suppl 2):63–70.

87. Ilfeld BM, Gearen PF, Enneking FK, et al. Total hip arthroplasty as an overnight-stay procedure using an ambulatory continuous psoas compartment nerve block: a prospective feasibility study. Reg Anesth Pain Med 2006;31(2):113–8.

88. Ilfeld BM, Ball ST, Gearen PF, et al. Ambulatory continuous posterior lumbar plexus nerve blocks after hip arthroplasty: a dual-center, randomized, triple-masked, placebo-controlled trial. Anesthesiology 2008;109(3):491–501.

89. Siddiqui ZI, Cepeda MS, Denman W, et al. Continuous lumbar plexus block provides improved analgesia with fewer side effects compared with systemic opioids after hip arthroplasty: a randomized controlled trial. Reg Anesth Pain Med 2007; 32(5):393–8.

90. Mauermann WJ, Shilling AM, Zuo Z. A comparison of neuraxial block versus general anesthesia for elective total hip replacement: a meta-analysis. Anesth Analg 2006;103(4):1018–25.

91. Choi PT, Bhandari M, Scott J, et al. Epidural analgesia for pain relief following hip or knee replacement. Cochrane Database Syst Rev 2003;(3): CD003071.

92. Andersen LJ, Poulsen T, Krogh B, et al. Postoperative analgesia in total hip arthroplasty: a randomized double-blinded, placebo-controlled study on peroperative and postoperative ropivacaine, ketorolac, and adrenaline wound infiltration. Acta Orthop 2007;78(2):187–92.

Anterior Hueter Approach in the Treatment of Femoro–Acetabular Impingement: Rationale and Technique

Cefin Barton, MB, BCh, MRCS(Ed), FRCS (Tr&Orth),
Kamaljeet Banga, MD, DNB(Ortho), Paul E. Beaulé, MD, FRCSC*

KEYWORDS

- Femoro-acetabular impingement • Hip arthroscopy
- Labral tear • Anterior approach • Young adult

In the last decade, femoro–acetabular impingement (FAI) has been recognized as a cause of pain and early arthrosis in the young adult hip.[1–3] Ganz and colleagues[1] described it and divided it into two main groups: CAM type presenting more commonly in young males, and pincer type more commonly in women in their late 30s or early 40s. CAM type impingement is defined as insufficient offset or concavity of the femoral head–neck junction causing shearing damage to the labral–chondral junction and acetabular articular cartilage. In pincer-type impingement, the primary deformity is on the acetabular side in the form of overcoverage (protrusio, coxa profunda, or acetabular retroversion) leading to abutment of the femoral neck against the acetabular rim, pinching the labrum between the femoral neck and the bony rim. It also typically causes a thin rim of acetabular articular cartilage damage. Although both types of deformities are found together in about 30% to 40% of hips,[4,5] recent evidence would suggest that presence of the CAM deformity, especially with alpha angles greater than 60°, is the driving deformity leading to hip pain.[5]

In 2009, the surgical correction of FAI deformity is an accepted treatment in patients presenting with hip pain with associated labral–chondral damage, with most recent series showing good-to-excellent results in over 80% of cases.[6–10] As with any surgical treatment, techniques will evolve to improve predictability of clinical outcome and minimize time to recovery and the risk of reoperation. More importantly, when one looks at the clinical results of FAI surgery, preservation of a healthy labrum appears to be a critical component of improved hip function after correction of the bony dysmorphism.[11] Some controversy remains, however as to how one should deal with the damaged chondro–labral junction, that is, isolated debridement versus labral takedown and refixation.[12] Currently, the senior author favors labral debridement and performs labrum takedown and refixation when the area of exposed subchondral bone underneath the delaminated acetabular cartilage flap is greater than 4 mm or when there is acetabular retroversion with a cross-over sign extending 10 mm beyond the acetabular roof.[3] In terms of surgical technique, it is clear that surgical dislocation of the hip joint will remain the most powerful tool in the surgeon's armamentarium.[13] It carries an inherent morbidity, however, in terms of risk of trochanteric nonunion and reoperation for painful internal fixation.[10,14] On the other hand, less-invasive techniques such as hip arthroscopy

Adult Reconstruction Unit, The Ottawa Hospital, University of Ottawa, 501 Smyth Road CCW 1646, Ottawa, ON, Canada
* Corresponding author.
E-mail address: pbeaule@ottawahospital.on.ca (P.E. Beaulé).

Orthop Clin N Am 40 (2009) 389–395
doi:10.1016/j.ocl.2009.03.002

are proving themselves to be as effective as open techniques,[15] but it is relatively more difficult to achieve a precise correction because of a limited field of view, which is why some have performed an anterior hip arthrotomy in conjunction with the arthroscopy to optimize visualization of the CAM deformity[16,17] (**Table 1**). Using this technique of combined hip arthroscopy to address the labral–chondral damage and Hueter anterior approach to correct the CAM deformity, Laude and colleagues reported good-to-excellent results in 78 out of 100 hips at a mean follow-up of 4.5 years, with 12 hips progressing to arthritis.

Historically, Carl Hueter first described the anterior approach in 1881 (see the article by Rachbauer and colleagues elsewhere in this issue); this approach was popularized by the Judet School for performing total hip arthroplasty. It uses the distal portion of the approach that many surgeons would recognize as the classical Smith Peterson approach, which is a muscle-splitting approach that uses a true internervous plane between the tensor fascia lata (TFL) and gluteus medius laterally (superior gluteal nerve) and sartorius and rectus femoris medially (femoral nerve). Letournel described a slight variation on the classical approach in 1980.[18] Instead of using the plane in between TFL and sartorius, the sheath of TFL is opened on its medial aspect, and

dissection to the deeper layer proceeds within this sheath to minimize damage to the lateral femoral cutaneous nerve. Although the experience with this technique remains limited, it permits one to:

- Completely preserve the capsule and Ligamentum teres while permitting efficient correction of the underlying bony deformity/dysmorphism
- Debride and repair the damaged labral–chondral junction
- Minimize surgical morbidity in respect to recovery time and risk of reoperation

Consequently, the authors began using this technique in early 2005 in patients who had a localized anterior deformity and for older female patients to minimize recovery time.

This article discusses the indications and diagnostic criteria and the surgical technique and early clinical results for the combined arthroscopic/ Hueter approach.

PATIENT SELECTION AND DIAGNOSTIC CRITERIA

Patients typically present as active people ranging in age from as young as 16 up to early 50s. The history is most commonly of an insidious onset of hip pain related to activity and in certain cases

Table 1
Advantages and disadvantages of the commonly used approaches to femoro–acetabular impingement

Approach	Advantages	Disadvantages
Surgical dislocation	Best visualization of head/neck junction Best visualization and access to acetabular rim Excellent intraoperative estimation of correction achieved Can be converted easily to a resurfacing[a]	Morbidity from trochanteric osteotomy: painful trochanteric fixation 1% of nonunion Large dissection Ligamentum teres disruption
Combined arthroscopic/Hueter	No dislocation preserves ligamentum and capsule Good, direct visualization of deformity[b] Intraoperative correction can be judged directly Minimally invasive Short surgical time Short recovery time	Not suitable for all deformities: coxa profunda, high riding greater trochanter Lateral cutaneous femoral nerve injury
Purely arthroscopic	Minimally invasive Short recovery time	Difficult to fully visualize deformity Partial capsulectomy often required

[a] If osteo-arthritis is advanced enough.
[b] As long as the deformity is in a position to which the Hueter window allows access.

related to a specific injury. The pain is typically in the midgroin area or referred to the buttock area, often localized by the patient by grasping the hip between thumb and index finger, the so-called C sign.[19] Patients often describe exacerbation of their pain after long periods of sitting or sporting activities with periods of rest from their activity providing them with some relief of pain. Recommencement, however, almost always is accompanied by a return of symptoms. Simple analgesics and anti-inflammatory medications are only partially effective. Physical examination often can be unremarkable apart from a limitation of internal rotation in flexion. Adduction of the hip in this position combined with internal rotation, the impingement test, also can reproduce their pain. A positive impingement test, however, must be taken in context with the history and imaging, as it is known to have a low kappa value in inter-rater reliability.[20]

Radiographic Investigation

Plain radiographs consist of an antero-posterior (AP) pelvis and a cross-table lateral or Dunn view of the affected hip[21] (**Fig. 1**). If there is loss of sphericity on the AP view, this typically will give one the pistol grip deformity.[4,22] Such a deformity can be more difficult to visualize through the Hueter anterior approach, because it tends to extend postero–laterally. The Dunn view is the most reproducible lateral view and also is known to be one of the best views for detecting a decreased head/neck offset.[23] The Dunn view is obtained with the patient lying supine, and an AP film is taken with the hip in 90° of flexion, neutral rotation, and 20° of abduction. The Alpha angle then is measured on the lateral radiograph (cross-table or Dunn view) (see **Fig. 1**).

MRI with gadolinium arthrography (MRA) is obtained with axial oblique (**Fig. 2**) and radial cut reconstructions (**Fig. 3**) using the femoral neck as the axis of rotation. These special views obtained on MRA provide valuable information in borderline cases (ie, alpha angle of 50° to 55° on the Dunn view) and are independent of patient position. In addition, the MRA provides information about the condition of the labrum and articular cartilage.

One must be careful how the radial reformats are interpreted comparatively to the axial oblique views when measuring the alpha angle. More importantly, as shown by Pfirrmann and colleagues,[22] the main location of the impinging CAM deformity lies between the 1 and 2 o'clock positions, making it accessible through the Hueter approach. Rakhra and colleagues[24] reported that in over 50% of cases, the radial reformat image gives an alpha angle value greater than 50° when compared with

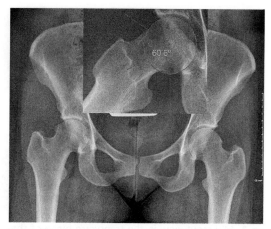

Fig. 1. AP pelvis and Dunn view radiograph showing loss of sphericity in the right hip. Inset shows Dunn view of the right with alpha angle of 60.6°.

the axial oblique. Because Notzli and colleagues[25] described the alpha angle on the axial oblique view, and others also have used this plane of measurement, it is unclear if the same cutoff or a larger one should be used for the radial reformats. The axial oblique slices are the views used routinely for managing these patients, as these are the current accepted standard.

RELATIVE CONTRAINDICATIONS

Relative contraindications include:

> Presence of coxa profunda or crossover sign extending 10 mm from the acetabular roof
> Femoral head/neck deformity extending postero laterally

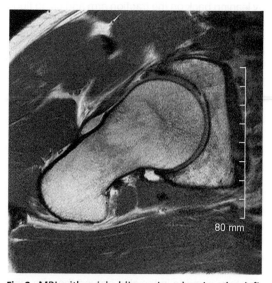

Fig. 2. MRI with axial oblique view showing the deficient concavity anteriorly.

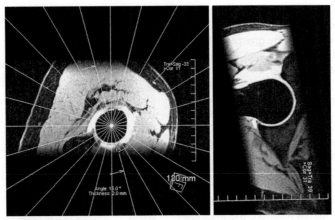

Fig. 3. MRI scout view in the transverse plane of the femoral neck showing the planes of the radial cuts. Inset showing radial cut image at the 1:30 position, where lack of concavity is quite dramatic.

Patients who have a high-riding greater trochanter requiring distal transfer such as in Legg-Calve-Perthes

Early joint space narrowing (1 mm to 2 mm) where joint arthroplasty may provide a more predictable outcome[12]

SURGICAL TECHNIQUE

The patient is positioned supine on regular fracture table. Arthroscopy of the hip is performed by placing a 10 in padded roll between the legs with both feet attached to traction boots.[26] Initially, some counter-traction is applied to the opposite leg, which is positioned in 20° to 30° of abduction. This prevents pelvic obliquity during the arthroscopy. Traction then is applied to the affected leg by leaning back on the traction arm and using fluoroscopy as a guide. Again, the leg is in 20° to 30° of abduction. Once one is happy that the hip is beginning to distract, the traction arm is locked, and the leg is adducted to a neutral position. Often a gentle pop can be heard as the hip looses its seal and distracts. Confirmation of adequate distraction is obtained by fluoroscopy. Care should be taken to have the foot slightly elevated from neutral on the traction post to give a few degrees of hip flexion. This prevents anterior subluxation of the hip during distraction and difficulty gaining access to the joint. The primary antero–lateral portal is placed superio–anterior to the tip of the greater trochanter. A spinal needle is advanced medially and caudally toward the dome of the femoral head as seen on fluoroscopy. Care should be taken to stay as close as possible to the head to avoid the portal traversing the labrum. A stab incision then is made in the skin around the wire, and a 5.0 mm trocar is advanced along the wire. The

trocar will be felt entering the joint, and at this point placement, is confirmed on fluoroscopy. The 70° angled scope then is introduced. The second portal (anterior) is placed along the line of the Hueter incision and later incorporated into it. This should be in line with the tip of the greater trochanter, and its entry point into the hip should be guided by direct vision from the scope. Once the two portals are established, the central compartment is inspected where labral and chondral damage can be assessed and treated as necessary (**Fig. 4**). Following arthroscopy, traction is released.

The planned Hueter incision then is made, incorporating the second arthroscopic portal. The anterior superior iliac spine (ASIS) is marked, as is the lateral edge of the patella. A line joining the two landmarks is drawn, and the 5 cm incision is parallel and 2 cm lateral to this line, starting proximally about 1 cm distal to the ASIS (**Fig. 5**). After dividing the subcutaneous fat, the TFL is identified and its sheath opened in line with the incision. Dissection proceeds within the sheath of TFL to avoid damage to the lateral femoral cutaneous nerve, which emerges either between TFL and sartorius or through the substance of sartorius. Once the deep surface of the sheath of TFL is breached, one will reach the innominate fascia in the interval between rectus femoris and gluteus medius. This is divided to reveal pericapsular fat. Also in this plane is the vastus lateralis, which signifies the distal limit of the dissection. The vastus is not dissected off the bone. The proximal landmark is the reflected head of rectus femoris intimately associated with the hip capsule. This can be divided and peeled medially to help reveal the white capsule of the hip. For treating FAI, however, this is unnecessary in most cases. An

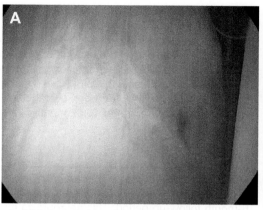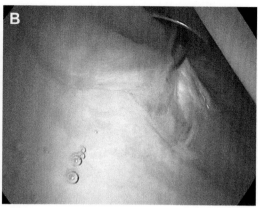

Fig. 4. (*A*) Intraoperative view of central compartment through the scope showing damaged labral chondral junction. (*B*) Intraoperative view after debridement of the damage.

incision then is made in the capsule of the hip in the line of the neck taking care not to damage the labrum at the proximal end of the arthrotomy (**Fig. 6**). The femoral head neck junction can be brought fully into the window created by gentle traction. The arthrotomy can be extended in a T shape along the acetabular rim and to enhance access, which also can be T'd at the intertrochanteric ridge if required. Again, care is taken not to damage the labrum. Rotation of the leg by the unscrubbed assistant permits proper visualization anteriorly and antero–laterally.

A high-speed burr then is introduced through the first arthroscopic portal (antero–lateral, **Fig. 7**) and used to remove the prominence and recreate the head neck offset. Bony debris is washed out, and the capsule is repaired. The patients are discharged on the day of surgery and restricted to 50% weight bearing for 3 weeks, at which time they are referred to a physical therapist. During those first 3 weeks, patients are encouraged to do stationary bike exercises.

CLINICAL RESULTS

The authors performed 24 combined hip arthroscopies with mini open anterior arthrotomies on 23 patients from September 2005 to December 2007. There were 5 men and 18 women, with average age 42.17 years (range 20 to 65 years). Out of 23 patients, 3 were lost to follow-up; 5 went on to reoperations, and the remaining 15 were followed for an average of 21.8 months (range 12 to 30 months). Their average Harris Hip Scores improved significantly from 70.23 (range 33 to 85) to 83.73 (range 47 to 99) ($P<.001$).

Case Presentation

A 31-year-old active woman presents with a 2-year history of insidious onset of right groin pain with difficulty with activities of daily living with increased pain with sporting activities. She has no history of trauma or childhood hip problems. Physical examination revealed a normal left hip. Internal rotation in flexion of the right hip was

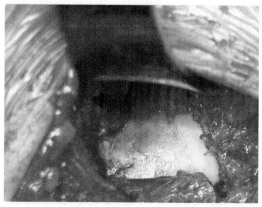

Fig. 5. Surface markings for arthroscopy (*crosses*) and planned Hueter incision.

Fig. 6. Intraoperative photograph of the head neck junction as seen through the Hueter window.

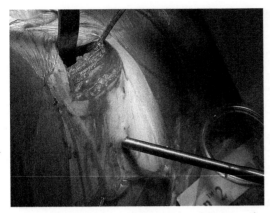

Fig. 7. Intraoperative photograph showing the introduction of a high-speed burr through the antero–lateral arthroscopic portal allowing good visualization of the burr tip and area of correction.

limited to 10° compared with 25° on the other side. The impingement test was positive. Plain radiographs demonstrated a spherical head with a CAM deformity on the Dunn view (see **Fig. 1**).

MRI arthrogram demonstrated a small labral tear at the 1 to 2 o'clock position with intact articular cartilage. The alpha angle measured 55° on the axial oblique and a maximum of 60° at the 3 o'clock position on the radial cuts. The authors felt she was a good candidate for the combined arthroscopic/Hueter approach. Her 6-month postoperative Dunn view is shown (**Fig. 8**), with an alpha angle now at 43.8°. Clinically, she has a greater range of motion and is pain-free.

Reoperations

There were five reoperations at a mean time of 15.2 months (range 4 to 22 months): one for intra-articular adhesions, three for correction of

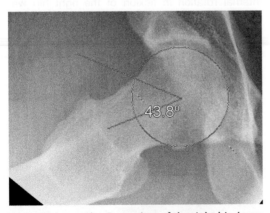

Fig. 8. Postoperative Dunn view of the right hip (same patient as **Fig. 1**) showing the correction achieved and restoration of the head/neck offset. Alpha angle illustrated.

mild dysplasia, and one for recurrent traumatic tear of the labrum. The one case of intra-articular adhesions is felt to be secondary to the use of bone wax on the exposed cancellous bone after recontouring of the head neck junction as reported by Beck.[27] Three cases with residual hip dysplasia had corrective surgery with a peri-acetabular osteotomy after an average of 16.67 months (range 15 to 18 months).

Complications

Lateral femoral cutaneous nerve injury
All were transient and made a full recovery by the 6-month follow-up period. This neuropraxia more than likely caused by the retraction used in obtaining exposure.

Ectopic ossification
We have encountered one case of myositis ossificans within the substance of tensor fascia lata.

SUMMARY

Overall, the authors have found this to be a very reliable, safe, and reproducible approach to treating FAI. The modification in the approach minimizes the risk of damage to the lateral femoral cutaneous nerve. The authors have come across some problems early in the use of the approach. It is important to appreciate where the head–neck junction is. Gentle traction will improve the view. If it is not recognized, then one risks burring into healthy normal head or burring too distal on the neck, leading to undercorrection. Once the arthrotomy has been performed and the head–neck junction is exposed, rotation of the leg is important to visualize all of the affected area. Again, failure to do this will lead to undercorrection.

REFERENCES

1. Ganz R, Parvizi J, Leunig M, et al. Femoroacetabular impingement: a cause for osteoarthritis of the hip. Clin Orthop Relat Res 2003;417:112–20.
2. Leunig M, Beaule PE, Ganz R. The concept of femoroacetabular impingement: current status and future perspectives. Clin Orthop Relat Res 2009; 467:616–22.
3. Beaule PE, Zaragoza EJ. Femoroacetabular impingement: diagnosis and treatment. In: Beaule PE, editor. The young adult with hip pain. Rosemont (IL): American Academy of Orthopaedic Surgeons; 2007. p. 63–74.
4. Beck M, Kalhor M, Leunig M, et al. Hip morphology influences the pattern of damage to the acetabular cartilage: femoroacetabular impingement as a cause

of early osteoarthritis of the hip. J Bone Joint Surg Br 2005;87:1012–8.

5. Allen DJ, Beaule PE, Ramadan O, et al. Prevalence of associated deformities and hip pain in patients with cam type femoroacetabular impingement. J Bone Joint Surg Br 2009;91:564–72.

6. Siebenrock KA, Schoeniger R, Ganz R. Anterior femoro–acetabular impingement due to acetabular retroversion. Treatment with periacetabular osteotomy. J Bone Joint Surg Am 2003;85:278–86.

7. Beck M, Leunig M, Parvizi J, et al. Anterior femoroacetabular impingement. Part II. Midterm results of surgical treatment. Clin Orthop Relat Res 2004; 418:67–73.

8. Murphy SB, Tannast M, Kim Y-J, et al. Debridement of the adult hip for femoroacetabular impingement. Indications and preliminary clinical results. Clin Orthop Relat Res 2004;429:178–81.

9. Larson CM, Giveans MR. Arthroscopic management of femoroacetabular impingement: early outcomes measures. J Arthroplasty 2008;24:540–6.

10. Beaule PE, LeDuff MJ, Zaragoza EJ. Quality of life outcome of femoral head/neck offset correction for femoroacetabular impingement. J Bone Joint Surg Am 2007;89:773–9.

11. Espinosa N, Rothenfluh D, Beck M, et al. Treatment of femoro-acetabular impingement: preliminary results of labral refixation. J Bone Joint Surg Am 2006;88:925–35.

12. Beaule PE, Allen DJ, Clohisy JC, et al. The young adult with hip impingement: deciding on the optimal intervention. J Bone Joint Surg Am 2009; 91:210–21.

13. Ganz R, Gill TJ, Gautier E, et al. Surgical dislocation of the adult hip. A new technique with full access to the femoral head and acetabulum without the risk of avascular necrosis. J Bone Joint Surg Br 2001;83: 1119–24.

14. Peters CL, Erickson JA. Treatment of femoro–acetabular impingement with surgical dislocation and debridement in young adults. J Bone Joint Surg Am 2006;88:1735–41.

15. Ilizaliturri V, Orcozo-Rodriguez L, Acosta-Rodriguez E, et al. Arthroscopic treatment of cam-type femoroacetabular impingement preliminary

report at 2 years minimum follow-up. J Arthroplasty 2008;23:226–34.

16. Laude F, Sariali E, Nogier A. Femoroacetabular impingement treatment using arthroscopy and anterior approach. Clin Orthop Relat Res 2009;467: 747–52.

17. Ribas M, Marin-Penna OR, Regenbrecht B, et al. Hip osteoplasty by an anterior minimally invasive approach for active patients with femoroacetabular impingement. Hip Int 2007;17:91–8.

18. Letournel E. Acetabular fractures: classification and management. Clin Orthop Relat Res 1980;151: 81–106.

19. Byrd JW. Hip arthroscopy: patient assessment and indications. Instr Course Lect 2003;52:711–9.

20. Martin RL, Sekiya JK. The interrater reliability of 4 clinical tests used to assess individuals with musculoskeletal hip pain. J Orthop Sports Phys Ther 2008; 38:71–7.

21. Clohisy JC, Carlisle JC, Beaule PE, et al. A systematic approach to the plain radiographic evaluation of the young adult hip. J Bone Joint Surg Am 2008;90: 47–66.

22. Pfirrmann CW, Mengiardi B, Dora C, et al. Cam and pincer femoroacetabular impingement: characteristic MR arthrographic findings in 50 patients. Radiology 2006;240:778–85.

23. Meyer DC, Beck M, Ellis T, et al. Comparision of six radiographic projections to assess femoral head/asphericity. Clin Orthop Relat Res 2006;445:181–5.

24. Rakhra K, Sheikh AM, Allen DJ, et al. Comparison of MRI alpha angle measurement planes in femoroacetabular impingement. Clin Orthop Relat Res 2009; 467:660–5.

25. Notzli HP, Wyss TF, Stoecklin CH, et al. The contour of the femoral head–neck junction as a predictor for the risk of anterior impingement. J Bone Joint Surg Br 2002;84:556–60.

26. Byrd JW. Arthroscopic management of hip pain. In: Beaule PE, editor. The young adult with hip pain. Rosemont (IL): American Academy of Orthopaedic Surgeons; 2007. p. 50–61.

27. Beck M. Groin pain after open FAI surgery: the role of intraarticular adhesions. Clin Orthop Relat Res 2009;467:769–74.

Gait and Motion Analysis of the Lower Extremity After Total Hip Arthroplasty: What the Orthopedic Surgeon Should Know

Mario Lamontagne, PhD[a,b,*], Mélanie L. Beaulieu, MSc[a],
Daniel Varin, BSc[a], Paul E. Beaulé, MD, FRCSC[c]

KEYWORDS

• Biomechanics • Kinematics • Kinetics • Hip • Gait • Motion

Human locomotion has been the subject of numerous publications over the last century. With the development of sequential photography (chronophotography) by Étienne-Jules Marey,[1] it was possible to capture animal and human movement and observe phenomena impossible to see with the naked eye. This made possible the first analyses of movement (ie, motion analysis). In the 1950s, the human locomotion in the cyclic fashion, called gait, was of large interest to assess the functional mobility of individuals.[2] From that point, gait analysis was considered an essential tool to assess the functional capacity of patients. **Motion analysis** refers to the analysis of a movement without taking into account the forces (eg, moments of force) that are generating this movement. **Gait analysis**, however, refers to the analysis of a particular type of movement—locomotion (eg, walking, running, stair ascending/descending)—and may (or may not) include the analysis of forces. Hence, a gait analysis can be a type of motion analysis. Moreover, **biomechanical analysis** is defined as an analysis of a movement and the forces producing the movement.

With the advancement of technology, a biomechanical analysis has evolved to include kinematics, kinetics, and muscle activity recordings.[3] A biomechanical analysis is the most comprehensive mean by which to quantify functional limitations. It allows clinicians to objectively assess the efficiency of treatments or the effectiveness of hip replacement approaches.[4] Given that more objective measurements of hip replacements are needed to assess the level of functionality of the hip joint after surgery, the orthopedic surgeon is highly encouraged to make use of the objective evidence provided by a biomechanical analysis.

ESSENTIAL COMPONENTS OF MOTION ANALYSIS
Gait Parameters

The motor development of human gait is a process that occurs over several years. Thereafter, gait patterns are fully integrated, and thus, gait parameters are constant and easy to compare between individuals. The efficiency of human gait depends on free joint mobility and muscular efficacy in timing and intensity.[5] Therefore, if there are any

This work was partly supported by Grant No. 82456 from the Canadian Institutes of Health Research.
[a] School of Human Kinetics, University of Ottawa, 125 University PVT, Ottawa, ON K1N 6N5, Canada
[b] Department of Mechanical Engineering, 161 Louis Pasteur, University of Ottawa, Ottawa, ON, Canada
[c] Division of Orthopaedic Surgery, The Ottawa Hospital, 501 Smyth Road, CCW 1646, Ottawa, ON K1H 8L6, Canada
* Corresponding author. School of Human Kinetics, University of Ottawa, 125 University PVT, rm 341, Ottawa, ON K1N 6N5, Canada.
E-mail address: mlamon@uottawa.ca (M. Lamontagne).

Orthop Clin N Am 40 (2009) 397–405
doi:10.1016/j.ocl.2009.02.001
0030-5898/09/$ – see front matter © 2009 Elsevier Inc. All rights reserved.

abnormalities in the functionality of lower-limb joints, it could be detected by the gait parameters. Those parameters can be measured by foot-switches,[6] accelerometers,[7] a pressure plate, or pressure insoles.[8] They can be useful to compare hip replacement patients to a healthy control group. However, the interpretation of the findings is limited to the overall changes in the gait, and conceals a potential compensation from adjacent joints of the lower limb or the contralateral lower limb. The measurement of gait parameters only represents the final outcome of the complex task of locomotion. It fails to provide information concerning force distribution, muscle timing and intensity, or coordination between segments. Results from studies that assess gait parameters can be used to merely extrapolate the causes of anomalies found in these parameters. Finally, measurement of gait parameters is limited to cyclic movements and cannot evaluate aperiodic movements, such as squatting.

Kinematics

Kinematics is defined as the study of motion without regard to the forces causing the motion. Variables of interest in human motion include linear and angular position, displacement, velocity, and acceleration. Early methods of observing those variables consisted of two-dimensional (2-D) chronophotography, for which manual processing was time consuming.[1] Modern automated motion capture systems now enable us to evaluate more people and to process data much faster. Most systems use skin markers to identify specific bony landmarks. And these systems are proficient at accurately capturing the positions of these markers. Since the markers are affixed to the skin to measure motion of the underlying bones, however, the movement of skin over bone (skin artifact) can translate into small errors in the calculation of the position of the joints' centers of rotation, and the position of the segments (eg, pelvis, thigh, and so forth).[9]

Kinematics provide more information than gait parameters because abnormalities can be identified for each articulation for each limb. This gives further information on which articulation exhibits an abnormal pattern compared with a normal population. However, since kinematics are only the observed motion, they do not reveal to us the causes of this abnormal motion. Stating that the activation pattern of a particular muscle (or muscle group) is causing the measured kinematic abnormality can only be a speculation and cannot be verified. To better understand the causes of

kinematic abnormalities, one must assess the forces acting at the joint by means of kinetics.

Kinetics

Kinetics refer to the forces causing movement. When they contract, muscles produce a linear force acting at a certain distance from a joint, which results in the generation of torque about that joint, and thus, movement. The kinetics explain this movement. To calculate joint-specific kinetics, an inverse dynamics approach is typically used. To use this approach, the body is firstly simplified as a rigid-linked, free-body model. Segments are considered rigid and articulate through frictionless joints. Then ground reaction forces (typically measured by force platforms) in combination with the movement of the limbs, are used to derive the resultant forces acting at the ankle, the knee, the hip, and so forth. Such a method gives important information on the force produced at each joint during a ballistic task. And we can subsequently infer muscle activation patterns that would result in the generation of those forces.

However, inverse dynamics does have its limitations. In reality, segments are not completely rigid; this is particularly true for the foot, where movement between the tarsal bones dissipates some energy, thus reducing the force transmitted to the ankle. Also, while the methods used for computing kinematics and kinetics use anthropometric measurements of the participants in their calculations, segment properties, such as moment of inertia and center of mass, and hip joint center calculations, are typically estimated from previous cadaveric studies, and therefore do not correspond exactly to the participants' anthropometry. Finally, data obtained from inverse dynamics only represent the net forces at each joint. Hence, it does not take into account the individual contribution of the different muscles acting at each joint.

Electromyography

Electromyography (EMG) can be used in conjunction with kinetic data to identify which muscles are activated, and at what intensity, when certain movements are produced. By comparing kinetic data with EMG data, one can identify the main contributors to a certain moment of force and can correlate abnormal kinetics with specific EMG abnormalities to identify dysfunctional muscles. This is of particular interest for physiotherapists in personalizing their rehabilitation programs.

Biomechanical Analysis: What to Look for?

With today's quantity of articles on the topic of biomechanics, the reader should know what makes one analysis better than another. Studies looking only at gait parameters can merely speculate on the causes of abnormal data. To explain the observed phenomena, one should perform a motion analysis to obtain kinematic data. With today's technology, researchers should not limit themselves to a 2-D analysis of movement. Although the movement of interest may occur mostly in one plane (eg, in the sagittal plane for the knee), movement in other planes is always present.[10] Researchers should always specify by what means kinematic data were obtained as it gives the reader an indication of the accuracy and validity of the data. Furthermore, a biomechanical analysis presenting kinetic, in combination with kinematic, data is considered a more complete evaluation of the patients' movement patterns, as it provides information on the forces causing the movements. Finally, a biomechanical analysis that combines kinematics, kinetics, and EMG can identify abnormal muscle activation patterns and correlate them with specific forces and kinematics abnormalities. This type of research is considered comprehensive, and thus, superior in quality. Also, studies looking at other articulations can provide insight into coordination between the segments—an important component of gait.

The presence of a control group is very important when performing a biomechanical analysis. The control group should be closely matched in age, height, and weight (or body mass index), given that the range of values for each kinematic, kinetic, or EMG variable in the general population is rather large, and therefore, abnormalities of the experimental group might go unnoticed. Caution must be observed with studies using the contralateral (or unaffected) limb as a control group because this limb's function could be altered to compensate for the affected limb.

MOTION ANALYSIS AND HIP ARTHROPLASTY

Murray and colleagues were among the first to report gait parameters and kinematics of walking for patients suffering from hip osteoarthritis (OA)[11] and for patients with a total hip arthroplasty.[12] They used 2-D chronophotography with an overhead mirror to measure lateral movement of the head. For OA participants, they observed several gait impairments considered as pain avoidance strategies, such as limited extension of the hip and ankle, limited knee flexion, greater pelvis anteversion, pelvis transverse rotation, lumbar flexion, and irregular movement of the head. The subjects, who were implanted with a McKee-Farrar prosthesis, showed improved function in 27 of the 30 cases.

Furthermore, kinetics have been used to compare total hip arthroplasty (THA) with hip resurfacing arthoplasty (HRA) in walking.[13] Mont and colleagues used three-dimensional (3-D) motion capture and force platforms to calculate the kinetics with an inverse dynamics approach. This study consisted of a verification of the calculated position of the hip joint center (HJC) by comparing it to pelvic x-rays. This ensured proper position of the HJC virtual marker within 1 cm from the actual HJC. In their study, subjects with HRA demonstrated normal hip abductor and extensor moments of force, unlike subjects with THA, at a mean of 13 months postsurgery.

Perron and colleagues[14] measured 3-D kinematics and kinetics, in conjunction with EMG of lower-limb muscles, of walking in women with THA who were compared with an age-, height-, and weight-matched healthy control group. They reported range of motion, moments, and powers of the hip, knee, and ankle joints. They considered the reduced hip extensor moment during early stance and the reduced range of hip extension during early push-up to be the most critical findings. They also observed prolonged activation of the gluteus maximus over the mid-stance period, suggesting that an increased passive resistance of the hip flexors, rather than muscle weakness, was responsible for the reduced hip extension.

More recently, Glaser and colleagues[15] measured kinematics (hip separation) and kinetics (hip-bearing contact forces) to compare two minimally invasive approaches (anterolateral and posterolateral) to a standard posterior approach. They used video fluoroscopy to measure hip separation while walking. They observed lower-hip separation and reduced hip forces for both minimally invasive approaches, indicating better performance for these approaches.

Consequently, researchers have been using gait and motion analyses for several decades as a valuable tool to assess functional recovery after surgery for patients with hip arthroplasty. With today's technology, researchers should be performing a comprehensive biomechanical analysis to quantify the presence of, or lack thereof, functional limitations. Such an analysis should take into account the forces acting at each joint to better understand how the movements are produced.

To demonstrate how a biomechanical analysis is performed and how to interpret the results, the following sections of this article will describe the methods and present kinematic and kinetic results of an ongoing study. The main objective is to report a biomechanical analysis of the hip joint of patients with THA ascending and descending stairs, and the interpretation of the findings that were compared with those of healthy matched participants. This article will also present critical issues related to the interpretation of biomechanical findings. By having a better knowledge of the use of the biomechanical analysis and the interpretation of the biomechanical outcomes, such an analysis can become a useful tool to guide the orthopedic surgeon in the selection of surgical approaches, and to measure the patient's physical limitations after the surgery.

MATERIALS AND METHODS
Participants

Twenty subjects with THA between the ages of 55 to 75 years old were recruited through the Ottawa Hospital, Division of Orthopaedic Surgery, on a voluntary basis. All were operated through a lateral approach (10 women and 10 men; age: 66.2 ± 6.7 y; BMI: 27.2 ± 5 kg/m^2). Exclusion criteria included bilateral hip replacement, hip replacement due to infection, fracture or failure of a previous prosthesis, concomitant surgical procedure during the surgery, and any past or present condition that could alter gait (ie, stroke). Twenty healthy control subjects (10 women, 10 men; age: 63.5 ± 4.4 y; BMI: 24.9 ± 3.5 kg/m^2) matched by age and BMI were recruited from the general population of the Ottawa region. Informed written consent, approved by the institutions' research ethics boards, was obtained from each participant.

Data Collection

Forty-five reflective markers of 14 mm in diameter strategically placed on the subjects were captured at 200 Hz with an infrared nine-camera motion analysis system (Vicon MX-13, Oxford Metrics, Oxford, UK) for 3-D joint angle calculation (**Fig. 1**). The motion capture system was calibrated according to the manufacturer's specifications. Up to four force plates (Model OR6-6-2000, AMTI, Watertown, MA; Model 9286AA, Kistler Instruments Corp, Winterhur, Swtz) recorded ground reaction forces at 1000 Hz. The AMTI force plates were embedded in a walkway flush with the flooring. The Kistler force plates were mounted on the first and second steps of a custom-built staircase, which consisted of three steps of 17.8 cm in height and 28.0 cm in depth, and handrails (see **Fig. 1**). The ground reaction forces, combined with the kinematic data, were used to calculate joint reaction forces, moments of force, and power.

Protocol

Upon arrival at the laboratory, the subjects were asked to change into tight-fitting clothes (shorts and t-shirt) that limit marker movement on the body, and to wear their own shoes. Height and weight of the subjects were noted and subsequently used in the model to calculate the joints' centers of rotation. The 45 reflective markers were placed on specific bony landmarks with Velcro on the clothes or double-sided tape applied on the skin. Firstly, the subjects performed a static trial in which they were asked to stand, and remain motionless, with their feet shoulder-width apart and arms in front parallel to the ground with their head up. Subsequently, they were instructed to ascend and descend the staircase without using the handrails, which were present for safety purposes, in a step-over-step manner. Three successful trials were recorded for each task from each subject for subsequent analyses.

Data Analysis

Kinematic data were obtained using Vicon's Nexus software (v1.2) and a custom-made model named University of Ottawa Motion Analysis Model. Based

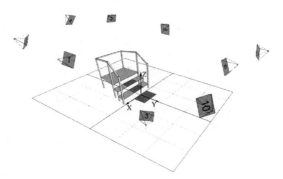

Fig. 1. 3-D camera setup with force plate position, custom-built staircase and global system of axis.

on the position of the skin markers, the model defined segments (eg, pelvis, femur) and calculated joint centers of rotation. Each segment had its own local coordinate system (relative to the global coordinate system) from which angles were calculated (**Fig. 2**). The static trial was used to determine the neutral angles in all planes. This method is based on the work of Davis III and colleagues.[16]

To measure the kinetics, an inverse dynamics approach is typically used. The human body is modeled as rigid segments linked with frictionless joints. The segments' mass and moments of inertia are estimated based on the work of Dempster.[17] The forces of muscles acting on a joint are reduced to a single resultant force. This reduction method is used to convert an undetermined set of equation to a determined one. Calculations are done from distal to proximal. Knowing the resultant force at the distal end of the segment, and the anthropometric properties, displacements, velocities, and accelerations of each segment, the net moments of force acting at each articulation can be calculated.

Joint power is obtained by the product of the net moment of force times the joint angular velocities. Joint power is the rate at which energy is generated or absorbed (concentric or eccentric work) at each articulation.

Data was normalized to 100% of the gait cycle (kinematics and kinetics) and body mass (kinetics). Trials were averaged for each task and for each group.

RESULTS AND DISCUSSION

The purpose of the present section is to provide an example of an interpretation of biomechanical (ie, kinematic and kinetic) findings. For this reason, only results relating to the hip joint are presented and discussed. However, it must be noted that it is important to evaluate a limb (eg, the leg) in its entirety given that the body is a linked system of interdependent segments.[13] The kinematics and kinetics of the joint of interest can be influenced by those of both the proximal and distal joints. Hence, one should focus on the contribution of all of the lower limb's joints (eg, hip, knee, and ankle) during a movement rather than solely focusing on an individual joint (eg, hip).

Stair Ascent

The THA group ascended the stairs in a different manner than did the control group, especially during the transition from double- to single-limb support phase. The majority of the hip kinematic and kinetic differences found between the groups were present at foot-off (FO) of the contralateral limb (ie, unoperated limb). Similar findings have been found by Foucher and colleagues.[18] As most of the body weight shifted on the ipsilateral hip (ie, operated limb), the control subjects produced a greater hip abduction moment of force while their hip was in a more adducted position, and generated more power, in comparison with the patients with THA (**Fig. 3**). We can speculate that activation of the gluteus medius, mainly responsible for hip abduction, produced this abduction moment of force to counteract an opposing moment produced by the individual's center of mass. And given that the lateral approach to THA does involve detachment (and repair) of the anterior third of the gluteus medius, and thus, a likely reduction in functionality, the

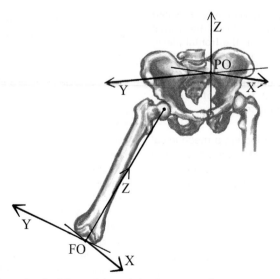

Fig. 2. Local coordinate systems (*xyz*) of the pelvis and the femur. FO, femur origin; PO, pelvis origin.

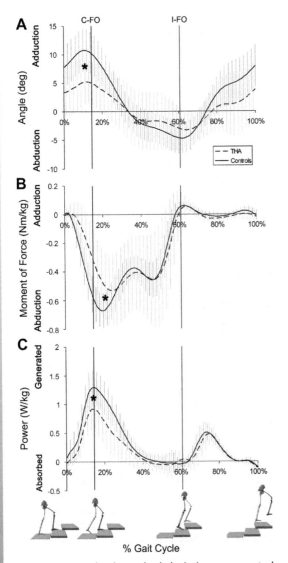

Fig. 3. Average (and standard deviation represented by gray vertical lines) (*A*) hip angle in the frontal plane, (*B*) hip moment of force in the frontal plane, and (*C*) net hip power during stair ascent, time-normalized to the gait cycle. The asterisks (*) represent statistically significant differences between the THA and control groups. C-FO, foot-off of contralateral limb; I-FO, foot-off of ipsilateral limb.

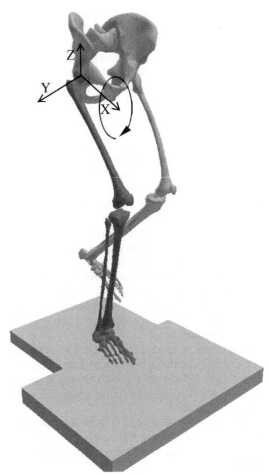

Fig. 4. Hip abduction moment of force depicted by the arrow around the x-axis of the hip's local coordinate system. This moment of force is required to avoid excessive hip adduction, and thus stabilize the pelvis in the frontal plane.

patients with THA may be adopting a mechanical strategy to ascend stairs that places the hip in this less adducted position; a position that requires a smaller counteracting hip abduction moment of force to stabilize the pelvis in the frontal plane (**Fig. 4**).

These are indeed speculations because this frontal plane moment of force calculated at the hip represents the net effect of all of the structures that produce this moment across the hip joint. Although we know that the main source of

generation of this moment of force are the abductor muscles (given that the forces produced by these muscles act at a distance from the center of a joint, thus producing a moment of force), these data do not provide any indication as to which individual muscles are contributing to this net moment. As a result, moments of force should be discussed without referring to specific anatomic structures (eg, gluteus medius). These kinetic data tell us the net effect of the structures, rather than their individual contributions. For these reasons, it can only be speculated that the smaller abduction moment of force observed as the patients with THA transitioned from double- to single-limb support resulted from a deficiency in the gluteus medius. We can, however, certainly conclude that in relation to the contribution of the hip adductors to the net frontal plane moment of force, the contribution of the hip abductors was greater. And that difference in contribution between the hip adductors and abductors—the net effect—was greater in the control subjects.

In the present example, the most plausible explanation would indeed be a reduction in hip abductor activation in the patients with THA. It has been demonstrated that frontal plane control of pelvic motion, achieved by the hip musculature, is critical to sustain total body balance including that of the upper body (ie, trunk, head, and arms) during level walking.[19] Specifically, the hip abductors are responsible for counteracting an adduction moment of force created by the force of gravity acting on the upper body's center of mass. The upper body creates this moment because its center of mass is located at a distance from the hip joint center (ie, when a force acts at a distance from the center of rotation, a moment of force is created). Hence, the patients with THA may be further tilting their pelvis and trunk laterally; which is an action that would shift the upper body's center of mass closer to hip joint center. The smaller hip adduction angle displayed by the THA group supports this explanation given that a lateral tilt of the pelvis decreases the adduction angle at the hip (**Fig. 3**A). If the center of mass of the upper body is acting at a closer distance from the hip joint center, a smaller adduction moment is generated, and therefore, a smaller counteracting moment of force needs to be generated by the hip abductors to achieve stability (**Fig. 3**B). In fact patients with THA display a deficiency in hip abductor recruitment, as assessed by EMG, during walking.[20]

Furthermore, as the power represents the product of the joint's net moment of force and angular velocity (as explained earlier in this article) or alternatively, the rate at which energy is generated (positive power or concentric work) or absorbed (negative power or eccentric work), it was not surprising that the control subjects ascended the staircase with greater generated power. The hip-joint power depicted in (**Fig. 3**C) represents the net effect of the powers in the sagittal, frontal, and transverse planes. However, the powers in the sagittal and frontal planes mostly contributed to this net power given the large magnitude of the moments of force in these planes in relation to the transverse plane moment. This is indeed predictable since the majority of the work is being performed in the sagittal plane to propel the body forward, and in the frontal plane to stabilize the pelvis and trunk as the subjects shifted their center of mass laterally at FO of the contralateral limb.

During this same transition from double- to single-limb support of the gait cycle in stair ascent, the control subjects displayed greater anterior and

superior hip joint reaction forces (**Fig. 5**). As with the moments of force, the joint reaction forces are the calculated, rather than directly measured, net forces which represent the net effect of all of the external and internal forces (eg, produced by the muscles, ligament, bone, and so forth) acting on the joint center. Hence, we cannot identify the exact structures that are responsible for the magnitude of the joint reaction forces. We do know, however, that these forces are highly dependent on those produced by the musculature surrounding the joint. These forces are not acting on the articular surface, but rather on the joint center. Consequently, these significantly smaller anterior and superior hip joint reaction forces calculated in the patients with THA represent a different hip-joint loading strategy, perhaps characterized by a consequential (to surgery) or deliberate deficiency in the recruitment of hip-joint muscles. This may be a strategy that these patients have adopted before the arthroplasty to

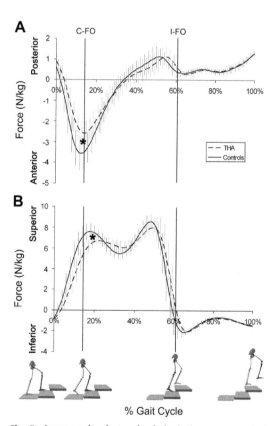

Fig. 5. Average (and standard deviation represented by gray vertical lines) (*A*) anterior-posterior and (*B*) inferior-superior hip joint reaction forces during stair ascent, time-normalized to the gait cycle. The asterisks (*) represent statistically significant differences between the THA and control groups. C-FO, foot-off of contralateral limb; I-FO, foot-off of ipsilateral limb.

reduce hip pain; which is a strategy that has become an adaptation of the neuromuscular system that may remain present postsurgery.[20] It may also be a result of the nature of the surgery given that the lateral approach of the THA involves the detachment of muscles important in hip stabilization.

Stair Descent

The THA group also descended the stairs in a different manner than did the control group. Because many biomechanical concepts were thoroughly explained earlier in this article, and that the main purpose of the present article is not to provide an exhaustive discussion of the results, but rather an explanation of their meaning and pertinence to orthopedics, this section provides a briefer examination of the results. The same biomechanical concepts will be illustrated but applied to the findings relating to stair descent.

As with stair ascent, the differences in stair ambulation strategies between groups were mostly present during the transition from double- to single-limb support phase (ie, FO of contralateral limb). As this transition occurred, the control subjects produced a greater hip internal-rotation moment of force while their hip was more externally rotated, in comparison with the patients with THA (**Fig. 6**). This indicates a greater net combined contribution of the hip internal and external rotators to the moment of force in the transverse plane in the control subjects. The hip internal rotators contributed to a greater extent of course, given that the net moment of force was one of internal rotation. Because the control subjects struck the ground with a more externally rotated hip (**Fig. 6A**), this group required a large hip internal-rotation moment to internally rotate the hip through the gait cycle. We could speculate as to why the THA group executed the foot strike portion of the cycle with a less externally rotated hip. We could speculate that it is a hip-joint stabilization strategy adopted by these subjects to compensate for a deficiency in hip musculature functionality. As mentioned, however, the present

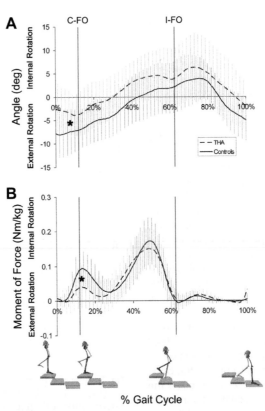

Fig. 6. Average (and standard deviation represented by gray vertical lines) (*A*) hip angle and (*B*) hip moment of force in the transverse plane during stair descent, time-normalized to the gait cycle. The asterisks (*) represent statistically significant differences between the THA and control groups. C-FO, foot-off of contralateral limb; I-FO, foot-off of ipsilateral limb.

article is not intended to provide an extensive discussion of the results.

Significant differences between the THA and control groups were also found for the hip joint reaction forces. Similar to the stair-ascent strategy adopted by the patients with THA, the latter descended the staircase with less anterior and superior joint reaction forces as FO of the contralateral limb occurred. This informs us that the patients with THA are using a stair descent strategy that is allowing them to significantly reduce loading at the prosthetic hip joint. Since hip joint reaction forces are highly dependent on the musculature surrounding the joint, we can conclude that this adopted strategy stems from a reduction in hip-joint muscle activation.

SUMMARY

A biomechanical analysis of human motion is a valuable tool to objectively quantify joint motion, and the forces producing this motion. However, one must remember what can be undoubtedly concluded from these findings, as opposed to what can be inferred. For example, joint reaction forces and moments of force tell us the net effect of all of the structures, including muscles, ligaments, and bones, among others, acting on the joint of interest. Conversely, it does not tell us the effect of a particular structure. Nevertheless, it remains that a combination of joint angles, reaction forces, moments of force, and powers provides us with information regarding the motion occurring at the joint, the general structures producing this motion, and the rate and nature of the work being done. This information constitutes a powerful tool that can be imperative to guide the orthopedic surgeon in the selection of surgical approaches, and to measure the patient's physical limitations postsurgery.

REFERENCES

1. Marey ÉJ. Le mouvement. Paris: G. Masson; 1894.
2. Eberhart HD, Inman VT. An evaluation of experimental procedures used in a fundamental study of human locomotion. Ann N Y Acad Sci 1951;51(7): 1213–28.
3. Delisa JA. Gait analysis in the science of rehabilitation. Darby (PA): Diane Publishing Co.; 1998.
4. Crowninshield RD, Johnston RC, Andrews JG, et al. A biomechanical investigation of the human hip. J Biomech 1978;11(1–2):75–85.
5. Perry J. Gait analysis: normal and pathological function. Thorofare (NJ): SLACK Inc; 1992.
6. Hausdorff JM, Ladin Z, Wei JY. Footswitch system for measurement of the temporal parameters of gait. J Biomech 1995;28(3):347–51.
7. Wiebren Z, At LH. Assessment of spatio-temporal gait parameters from trunk accelerations during human walking. Gait Posture 2003;18(2):1–10.
8. Webster KE, Wittwer JE, Feller JA. Validity of the GAITRite walkway system for the measurement of averaged and individual step parameters of gait. Gait Posture 2005;22(4):317–21.
9. Benoit DL, Ramsey DK, Lamontagne M, et al. In vivo knee kinematics during gait reveals new rotation profiles and smaller translations. Clin Orthop Relat Res 2007;454:81–8.
10. Kowalk DL, Duncan JA, Vaughan CL. Abduction adduction moments at the knee during stair ascent and descent. J Biomech 1996;29(3):383–8.
11. Murray MP, Gore DR, Clarkson BH. Walking patterns of patients with unilateral hip pain due to osteoarthritis and avascular necrosis. J Bone Joint Surg Am [series A] 1971;53(2):259–74.
12. Murray MP, Brewer BJ, Zuege RC. Kinesiologic measurements of functional performance before and after McKee-Farrar total hip replacement. A study of thirty patients with rheumatoid arthritis, osteoarthritis, or avascular necrosis of the femoral head. J Bone Joint Surg Am 1972;54(2):237–56.
13. Mont MA, Seyler TM, Ragland PS, et al. Gait analysis of patients with resurfacing hip arthroplasty compared with hip osteoarthritis and standard total hip arthroplasty. J Arthroplasty 2007;22(1):100–8.
14. Perron M, Malouin F, Moffet H, et al. Three-dimensional gait analysis in women with a total hip arthroplasty. Clin Biomech (Bristol, Avon) 2000;15(7): 504–15.
15. Glaser D, Dennis DA, Komistek RD, et al. In vivo comparison of hip mechanics for minimally invasive versus traditional total hip arthroplasty. Clin Biomech (Bristol, Avon) 2008;23(2):127–34.
16. Davis RB III, Õunpuu S, Tyburski D, et al. A gait analysis data collection and reduction technique. Hum Mov Sci 1991;10(5):575–87.
17. Dempster WT. Space requirements of the seated operator. Technical report WADC-TR-55-159. Dayton (OH): Wright-Patterson Air Force Base; 1995.
18. Foucher KC, Hurwitz DE, Wimmer MA. Do gait adaptations during stair climbing result in changes in implant forces in subjects with total hip replacements compared to normal subjects? Clin Biomech (Bristol, Avon) 2008;23(6):754–61.
19. MacKinnon CD, Winter DA. Control of whole body balance in the frontal plane during human walking. J Biol 1993;26(6):633–44.
20. Vogt L, Banzer W, Pfeifer K, et al. Muscle activation pattern of hip arthroplasty patients in walking. Res Sports Med 2004;12(3):191–9.

Spatiotemporal Parameters of Gait After Total Hip Replacement: Anterior versus Posterior Approach

Nicola A. Maffiuletti, PhD[a], Franco M. Impellizzeri, MS[a],
Katharina Widler, MS[a], Mario Bizzini, MS, PT[a],
Michael S.H. Kain, MD[b], Urs Munzinger, MD[c],
Michael Leunig, MD[c],*

KEYWORDS

- Walking ability • Hip arthroplasty • Surgical technique
- Stiffness • Pain

Multiple surgical approaches have been described for total hip arthroplasty (THA) and each one has advantages and disadvantages. The posterior approach, although the most commonly used approach, can be associated with a high rate of hip dislocation ranging from 1% to 10%.[1–4] The anterolateral and the direct anterior approaches were described in part to help prevent dislocations. There is an increased interest in the direct anterior approach for THA because it is thought to be a more muscle sparing procedure allowing for excellent exposure of the acetabulum and a low dislocation rate.[5,6] The negative aspects of this approach are that it is technically difficult, specialized equipment is needed, and damage to the tensor fascia latae (TFL) and rectus femoris muscles can occur.[5,7]

Arthritis outcome scores, dislocation rates, and radiographic analysis are commonly used modalities to assess the clinical success of arthroplasty,[8–10] yet little literature has compared the multiple surgical techniques for THA in terms of objective function (eg, gait analysis). Few studies have compared the posterior and the direct anterior approaches leaving a void in the current literature as to how these approaches compare.[7,11] In a cadaveric evaluation of the muscle damage between the two approaches, Meneghini and colleagues[7] reported similar muscle damage overall with both approaches, with the greatest difference between approaches occurring in the gluteus minimus, and no difference for the gluteus medius muscle. The gluteus minimus had 18% of its muscular area injured and 23% of the tendons surface area damaged in the posterior approach compared with 8.5% and 4.6% respectively for the direct anterior approach. Nakata and colleagues[11] compared these two approaches and reported that 34% of subjects in direct anterior approach group were able to ambulate without assistive devices 3 weeks after THA compared with 19% of subjects in the posterior approach group. Additionally, they reported a significant increase in walking velocity during a 50-m test in the direct anterior group at 2 months postoperatively, but no objective gait analysis was performed. To our knowledge, only Ward and colleagues[12] compared spatiotemporal walking parameters between these two approaches, however they used a body-mounted accelerometry system which suffers from some methodological limitations[13] leading to inaccurate assessments of speed and step length.

[a] Neuromuscular Research Laboratory, Schulthess Clinic, Lengghalde 2 - 8008 Zurich, Switzerland
[b] M.E. Müller Foundation North America, Schulthess Clinic, Lengghalde 2 - 8008 Zurich, Switzerland
[c] Lower Extremity Unit, Schulthess Clinic, Lengghalde 2 - 8008 Zurich, Switzerland
* Corresponding author.
E-mail address: michael.leunig@kws.ch (M. Leunig).

Orthop Clin N Am 40 (2009) 407–415
doi:10.1016/j.ocl.2009.02.004

The main aim of this preliminary study was to compare gait characteristics following THA surgery between subjects operated by way of a direct anterior approach and a posterior approach. Walking variables of these subjects were also compared with a group of age-matched healthy individuals. Since hip-abductor muscles, which play a crucial role during the stance phase of gait, are damaged to a greater extent with the posterior approach,[7] we hypothesized the use of a posterior approach for THA would result in a greater gait impairment when compared with the anterior approach.

MATERIALS AND METHODS
Subjects and Experimental Procedures

Subjects were randomly selected from postoperative lists and medical files of the Schulthess Clinic (Zurich, Switzerland). Fourteen women and twenty men with a diagnosis of primary osteoarthritis of the hip were identified and volunteered to participate in the study. Subjects were allocated to the anterior or posterior groups, according to the THA surgical approach. All posterior approaches were performed by a senior surgeon (UM) who has performed more than 2500 THA using the posterior procedure, and all anterior approaches were performed by another senior surgeon (ML) who has performed more than 250 THA using the anterior procedure. All subjects had to be able to ambulate without assistive devices and be available for gait assessments approximately 6 months postoperatively (mean follow-up 6.2 ± 0.4 months). Subjects were excluded if they suffered from any disease, disorder, or behavior affecting the function of the uninvolved limb. A control group of 17 healthy subjects matched for sex, age, and body mass was also tested. Testing consisted of radiographic assessment, outcome questionnaires, and spatio-temporal gait analysis. All subjects consented before participation, the study was conducted according to the Declaration of Helsinki, and the local ethical committee approved the protocol.

Surgical Procedures

The anterior approach for THA, first described by Judet and Judet in 1949 uses the interval between the TFL and the sartorius.[14,15] The anterior approach in this series was performed with the patient supine, on a regular operating room table with both lower extremities prepped out and included in the field. A straight 8- to 10-cm incision starting 2 cm lateral and distal to the anterior superior iliac spine and the fascia of the TFL is opened anteriorly. To protect the lateral femoral cutaneous nerve, the incision is kept slightly lateral to the interval between the TFL and sartorius. The TFL is dissected off the intramuscular septum and retracted laterally. The sartorius is retracted medially to expose the rectus femoris. The deep fascia of the TFL is incised and the plane between the capsule and the rectus femoris is developed with a Cobb elevator. An eva retractor is then placed into this interval to retract the rectus femoris and sartorius medially. The indirect head of the rectus femoris can be transected if exposure is not adequate. The gluteus medius, gluteus minimus, and TFL are retracted laterally to expose the hip capsule with a second eva retractor. After capsulectomy and femoral neck osteotomy the acetabulum is exposed and reaming can begin for acetabular component placement. The patients' legs are then placed in the figure-of-four position, with the operative hip extended and the femur externally rotated to expose the femoral canal. A press-fit or cemented femoral component can be used with this approach. Once the components are in, a Hemovac drain is placed, the wound is thoroughly irrigated and a three-layer closure is performed. The fascia of the TFL is closed with a running absorbable suture. The subcutaneous tissue is then closed with interrupted absorbable sutures and the skin is closed also with a running monocryl. The drain remains in from 24 to 48 hours.

The posterior approach was performed with patients in the lateral position. A 10- to 15-cm incision is made in line with the posterior femur and gently curved posteriorly at the tip of the greater trochanter. The fascial layer is split in addition to the gluteus maximus. Once the gluteus maximus is split, the bursa over the greater trochanter is incised and retracted posteriorly. The leg is externally rotated and the piriformis and external rotators are identified. The external rotators and posterior capsule are incised and reflected posteriorly. At this point the femoral head is dislocated and with more external rotation. The lesser trochanter is identified and a femoral neck osteotomy is performed. The acetabulum is exposed with retractors on the either side of the anterior and posterior walls. Acetabulum is then exposed fully for reaming. The femur is exposed with an assistant holding the leg in internal rotation. Again, a cemented or press-fit stem can be implanted. Once the components are in place the wound is irrigated and the capsule and external rotators are repaired to the posterior trochanter with several transosseus sutures. The fascial sheet, subcutaneous tissue, and skin are closed with absorbable suture. At the end of THA surgery, two drains are positioned for 24 hours.

Both posterior and anterior subjects were discharged once cleared by each respective surgeon.

The total length of hospital stay was around 7 days for the anterior approach and about 12 days for the posterior approach. Subjects received gait training with crutches, taught isometric exercises following surgery, and instructed to perform these exercises on their own. Rehabilitation guidelines were given to the subjects after discharge from the clinic and included weight bearing as tolerated, pool and range of motion exercises, generic strengthening and balance exercises (see Trudelle-Jackson and Smith[16]). Subjects were advised to complete two rehabilitation sessions per week (duration approximately 30 minutes) for 4 to 6 weeks, under the supervision of a qualified physical therapist. All subjects answered a rehabilitation questionnaire before performing the functional tests: 60% of the subjects participated in physical therapy sessions (10 out of 17 in the anterior group and 11 out of 17 in the posterior group), while the remaining 40% performed exercises at home and without direct supervision.

Radiographic Assessment

Radiographic assessment was performed using the anteroposterior pelvis and lateral radiograph corresponding to the clinical visit associated with the gait analysis. The anteroposterior pelvis was used to evaluate acetabular cup inclination (abduction angle) and for any leg length discrepancy. The lateral radiograph was used to evaluate acetabular cup anteversion. Both the anteroposterior and lateral radiographs were used to assess the presence of ectopic bone formation according to the Brooker and colleagues[17] classification.

Self-Reported Questionnaires

Subjects completed two self-administered questionnaires: the Western Ontario and McMaster Universities (WOMAC) Osteoarthritis Index, and the Short-Form 12-Item Health Survey (SF-12). The WOMAC is a disease-specific questionnaire used to measure symptoms and physical function disability. By using Likert scales, its 24 items probe three patient-relevant dimensions: pain (five items), stiffness (two items), and physical function (17 items). Scores range from 0 to 20 (pain), 0 to 8 (stiffness) and 0 to 68 (function). For clarity, however, the scores of the three dimensions were converted to a 0 to 100 scale, where 100 indicates the worst possible state. In the present study, the valid and reliable German version of WOMAC was used.[18] The SF-12 is a self-administered generic measure of quality of life.[19] Scores were transformed into two weighted summary scores for physical function (physical component) and mental health (mental component). The higher the score the better the health state and vice versa. The scores of the two components were standardized in relation to the United States population (mean: 50, SD: 10).[20]

Spatiotemporal Gait Analysis

Spatiotemporal parameters of gait were measured with the use of an electronic mat (GAITRite, CIR Systems Inc. Clifton, NJ, USA), which has been shown to provide valid and reliable data.[21,22] The instrumented mat used in this study (thickness 6 mm; total length 823 cm) has an active sensor area of 732 cm long and 61 cm wide. The active area contains 27,648 pressure sensors arranged in a grid pattern with a spatial resolution of 1.27 cm and a sampling frequency of 80 Hz.

Subjects wore a comfortable pair of flat-soled walking shoes. Each individual was required to walk at two different speeds: self-selected comfortable ("walk at a pace that is comfortable for you") and fast ("walk at a pace that is faster than you would normally walk"). Before data collection subjects practiced walking over the mat at both velocities to familiarize themselves with testing procedures. Each trial began and ended approximately 2 m from the mat so that a constant gait pattern was maintained. Three trials were recorded for each subject and for each speed, and the average was used for subsequent analysis.

Data from the activated sensors was collected by a series of on-board processors and transferred to a personal computer by way of an interface cable. A dedicated software (GAITRite Gold, Version 3.2b, CIR Systems Inc. Clifton, NJ, USA) was used to process the data into footfall patterns and to calculate the following gait parameters: walking speed (m/s), cadence (steps/min), step and stride lengths (cm), stance and swing phase durations (ms), single and double support durations (percentage of gait cycle), heel-heel support distance (cm) and toeing out (degrees). For subjects with THA, only the data for the operated limb were retained. For control subjects, left and right limb data were averaged together. These spatiotemporal variables are classically used in gait analysis studies with orthopedic populations.[12,23,24]

Statistical Analysis

After check for normality, differences in subject characteristics, radiographic outcomes, questionnaire outcomes, and gait parameters between groups (anterior, posterior, control) were examined using a one-way ANOVA (subject characteristics), an unpaired Student's *t*-test (radiographic outcomes), a Friedman's test (questionnaire outcomes) or a one-way ANCOVA with sex as a covariate (gait parameters). If significant main effect was present, a Fisher's LSD post hoc test was conducted. The significance level was set at $P<.05$ for all analyses. Effect sizes[25] were also calculated for each gait parameter comparison (anterior versus posterior groups).

RESULTS
Subject Demographics

Each group consisted of 17 subjects with 10 males and 7 females (**Table 1**). All subjects were approximately 69 years of age with similar height and body mass. There was no statistical difference between controls and the experimental groups. All acetabular components were press-fit. There were two cemented femoral components and 32 press-fit components.

Radiographic Outcomes

Cup inclination, cup anteversion and leg-length discrepancy did not differ significantly between the anterior (43.1 ± 3.5°, 24.0 ± 5.7° and 0.17 ± 4.09 mm) and posterior (44.1 ± 3.9°, 25.8 ± 6.2° and 0.31 ± 4.38 mm) groups. One anterior subjects and one posterior subject had ectopic bone formation classified as grade 2. One anterior and two posterior subjects had grade 1 ectopic bone formation, while the remaining subjects had no ectopic bone formation (grade 0).

Questionnaire Outcomes

WOMAC pain and function scores, and SF-12 physical and mental components, did not differ significantly between anterior, posterior, and control groups (**Table 2**), contrary to WOMAC stiffness score (Chi^2 = 8.667; $P = .013$), which was significantly higher in the posterior compared with anterior ($P<.05$) and control ($P<.001$) groups.

Gait Parameters

At self-selected walking speed, no significant main effect of group was observed for the different spatiotemporal gait variables (**Figs. 1**A and **2**A, **Table 3**). At fast speed, several interesting group differences were observed. Walking velocity was significantly lower for the anterior ($P = .005$) and posterior ($P = .044$) groups than for healthy controls (**Fig. 1**B). Similarly, both step (**Fig. 2**B) and stride lengths were significantly shorter for THA patients ($P<.05$), irrespective of the approach, compared with their healthy counterparts. All the other spatiotemporal parameters did not differ significantly between the anterior, posterior and control groups (**Table 4**). For the different gait parameters, effect sizes were trivial (<0.2) to small (0.2–0.5).

DISCUSSION

Several findings were observed in the present preliminary study: (1) both anterior and posterior procedures provided excellent outcome for pain and function, which was comparable to healthy controls; (2) irrespective of THA surgical approach for primary osteoarthritis, subjects demonstrated an impaired walking performance (lower velocity, shorter step and stride lengths) during an accelerated walking speed but not at self-selected speed compared with healthy controls; (3) posterior approach subjects reported higher stiffness scores using the WOMAC questionnaire, compared with the anterior subjects.

Based on a recent cadaveric study documenting greater muscle damage of the gluteus minimus with the posterior than with the anterior THA surgical procedure,[7] we hypothesized the former approach would result in a greater walking impairment compared with the latter. The gluteus minimus is an essential contributor of the stance phase of gait which is the best index of the limb's support capacity.[26] Hip abductor activation begins

| Table 1 |
| Subject characteristics by group[a] |

	Anterior (n = 17)	Posterior (n = 17)	Control (n = 17)
Male (n)	10	10	10
Female (n)	7	7	7
Age (years)	68 (6)	69 (5)	69 (4)
Height (cm)	166 (9)	168 (6)	169 (10)
Body mass (kg)	71 (11)	77 (15)	73 (11)
BMI (kg/m^2)	25.6 (3.3)	27.2 (4.2)	25.5 (2.7)

[a] Mean values (SD).

Table 2
Questionnaire outcomes by group[a]

		Anterior	Posterior	Control
WOMAC pain (0–100)	↑ worst ↓ best	0 (2.5)	0 (12.5)	0 (2.9)
WOMAC stiffness (0–100)	↑ worst ↓ best	0 (12.5)[b]	12.5 (37.5)	0 (6.3)[b]
WOMAC function (0–100)	↑ worst ↓ best	4.4 (8.8)	2.9 (21.3)	0 (2.9)
SF-12 physical component[c]	↓ worst ↑ best	54.8 (7.6)	50.3 (15.4)	55.2 (4.4)
SF-12 mental component[c]	↓ worst ↑ best	58.8 (2.8)	58.6 (9.4)	57.8 (3.3)

[a] Median values (interquartile range).
[b] Significantly lower than posterior ($P<.05$).
[c] Standardized scores (United States population, mean: 50, SD: 10).[20]

at the end of the terminal swing and the intensity of this action quickly increases to approximately 20% of maximal activation, with a peak immediately following initial contact and persists through mid stance.[27] However, we observed no significant difference between the posterior and anterior groups in spatiotemporal gait parameters, including stance duration, probably because of the possible damage to the TFL with the anterior procedure,[7] another abductor muscle activated during the initial half of stance.[27] On the other hand, the occurrence of rectus femoris damage with the anterior technique, and not with the posterior technique,[7] would not translate into sizeable gait alterations, because of the inconsistent participation of this hip flexor/knee extensor muscle during free walking.[26]

Irrespective of the THA group, subjects walked at a significantly slower velocity (-8%) and using significantly shorter steps (-6%) compared with their healthy peers, but only when they were asked to walk at a faster than normal velocity. As previously reported for subjects with total knee arthroplasty,[28] these abnormalities in walking patterns,

which can last for several years after surgery, occurred despite excellent clinical and radiographic scores. On the other hand, no significant group differences were observed at the self-selected comfortable walking speed, and all subjects were able to increase their speed by 28% when they were asked to walk at a faster than normal velocity, similar to the increase observed in healthy individuals (+32%). Such ability to modulate walking speed, which was obtained by simultaneously increasing stride length (13%) and cadence (15%), could be viewed as an important functional outcome, particularly in relation to safety and pain. Failure to increase stride length would indeed have functional consequences, such as altered balance control, which could, in turn, increase patients' risk of falling.[29] In the same way, patients with knee pain increase their walking speed by increasing the cadence and not the step length,[30] contrary to the subjects tested in this study.

Walking speed is an indicator of lower-limb function in orthopedic patients.[31] Its assessment is safe, simple (even with low technology

Table 3
Spatiotemporal gait parameters at self-selected speed by group[a]

	Anterior	Posterior	Control	$F_{(2,47)}$; P^b
Cadence (steps/min)	114.7 (8.3)	116.7 (8.0)	116.2 (6.3)	0.36; 0.701
Stride length (cm)	141.0 (14.6)	142.4 (14.2)	149.0 (7.9)	2.70; 0.077
Stance (ms)	653 (50)	635 (53)	634 (43)	0.92; 0.407
Swing (ms)	398 (33)	396 (27)	403 (17)	0.36; 0.701
Single support (%)	38.2 (1.0)	38.5 (1.3)	38.9 (1.3)	1.64; 0.204
Double support (%)	23.9 (2.0)	23.1 (2.9)	22.3 (2.4)	1.85; 0.168
Heel-heel support (cm)	8.8 (1.8)	9.2 (2.8)	7.9 (2.3)	1.41; 0.254
Toeing out (°)	5.9 (4.0)	7.2 (4.7)	6.9 (4.1)	0.42; 0.660

[a] Mean values (SD).
[b] One-way ANCOVA results.

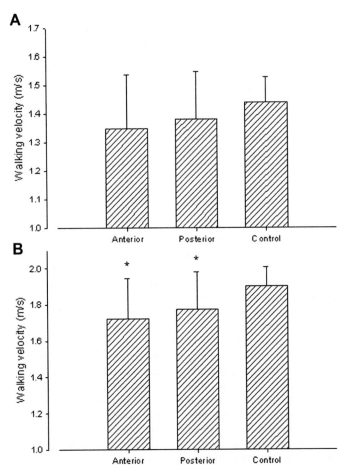

Fig. 1. Walking velocity at normal (*A*) and fast (*B*) speeds by group. Mean values and SD. *Significantly lower than control (*P*<.05).

equipment) and respects the specificity of daily living, in particular when subjects are required to walk using different instructions (normal, fast, slow) and conditions (up/downhill, different surfaces, with/without weights, and so forth). In the present study, we provide some evidence for the construct validity of this parameter, by showing that patients with THA selected a slower, faster than normal velocity compared with their age-matched controls. In addition, recent studies using similar subjects and methodologies demonstrated that self-selected gait velocity declines from 1 m/s preoperatively to 0.28 m/s 2 days postoperatively, and increases again to 1.07, 1.14 and 1.28 m/s, at 6 weeks, 3 months, and 6 months after THA surgery.[12,32–34] Additionally, as a methodological recommendation, our results suggest that assessment of walking parameters at faster than normal velocity, in addition to the self-selected comfortable velocity, is required for comparisons between subjects and healthy controls.

In the last few years, differences in spatiotemporal gait parameters between multiple surgical approaches (eg, long posterior, posterior, anterior, 2-incision, anterolateral, posterolateral) in patients with THA have been investigated using different methodologies and technologies (eg, force plates, high-speed cameras, body-mounted accelerometers).[12,33,34] However, none of these studies were capable of detecting significant differences in gait parameters between surgical approaches, from 6 weeks to 3 months postoperatively. Paradoxically, no difference was observed even between short-incision, including hip resurfacing,[35] and long-incision THA surgeries,[12,32,36] probably because the amount of muscle damage is essentially the same for these procedures.[37] Our results corroborate these findings, and further indicate that the surgical technique allowing better recovery of walking function after THA is far from being determined.

One limitation of our study is that it was a cross-sectional study, meaning causal conclusions were

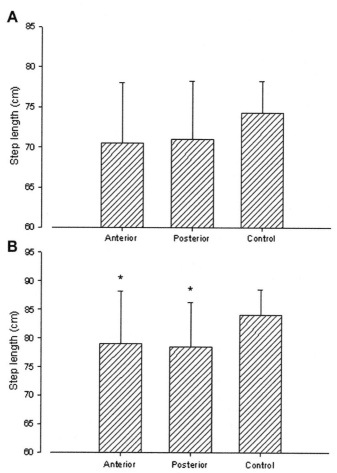

Fig. 2. Step length at normal (*A*) and fast (*B*) speeds by group. Mean values and SD. *Significantly lower than control (*P*<.05).

not allowed. We did not control for preoperative walking status, which has been shown to be, together with patient age, a potential predictor of postoperative walking speed.[12] In the same way,

we did not verify that the two subject groups had similar levels of activity preoperatively, which could have confounded, at least partly, the present findings. On the other hand, we included a group

Table 4
Spatiotemporal gait parameters at fast speed by group[a]

	Anterior	Posterior	Control	$F_{(2,47)}$; P^b
Cadence (steps/min)	130.4 (9.9)	134.8 (10.6)	136.2 (8.4)	2.14; 0.129
Stride length (cm)	158.9 (18.1)[c]	158.7 (15.2)[c]	168.3 (9.0)	3.96; 0.026
Stance (ms)	562 (48)	540 (47)	530 (36)	2.78; 0.073
Swing (ms)	363 (25)	357 (27)	354 (21)	0.63; 0.535
Single support (%)	39.9 (1.3)	39.6 (1.6)	40.1 (1.2)	0.46; 0.632
Double support (%)	20.9 (2.4)	20.5 (3.0)	19.9 (2.2)	0.54; 0.585
Heel-heel support (cm)	9.1 (1.8)	9.7 (2.8)	8.2 (2.7)	1.66; 0.201
Toeing out (°)	5.7 (4.0)	6.7 (5.2)	5.8 (3.7)	0.24; 0.789

[a] Mean values (SD).
[b] One-way ANCOVA results.
[c] Significantly lower than control (*P*<.05).

of healthy controls matched for sex, age, and body mass, and we conducted our study at a time when muscle damage repair and bone healing have generally occurred[12] (ie, 6 months after surgery) to minimize their influence on walking parameters. Effect sizes were trivial to small, suggesting low probability of type II error, and sample size was similar to the only study having compared gait parameters between subjects with anterior and posterior THA.[12]

This is a preliminary study. The obtained results will be used to design randomized controlled trials aimed at determining which surgical approaches produce better functional recovery following THA surgery. Once gait impairments associated with the multiple surgical approaches are clearly recognized, the effectiveness of classical and innovative rehabilitation procedures (pre- and postoperative) will be experimentally compared in an attempt to optimize patient care and safety.

SUMMARY

Six months after THA surgery, gait characteristics were comparable between subjects having received the direct anterior approach and the posterior approach, despite excellent clinical and radiographic scores. Subjects operated with the posterior approach reported significantly higher stiffness than anterior subjects, but similar pain and function was reported.

REFERENCES

1. Berry DJ, von Knoch M, Schleck CD, et al. The cumulative long-term risk of dislocation after primary Charnley total hip arthroplasty. J Bone Joint Surg Am 2004;86-A(1):9–14.

2. Heithoff BE, Callaghan JJ, Goetz DD, et al. Dislocation after total hip arthroplasty: a single surgeon's experience. Orthop Clin North Am 2001;32(4):587–91, viii.

3. Khan RJ, Fick D, Khoo P, et al. Less invasive total hip arthroplasty: description of a new technique. J Arthroplasty 2006;21(7):1038–46.

4. Peters CL, McPherson E, Jackson JD, et al. Reduction in early dislocation rate with large-diameter femoral heads in primary total hip arthroplasty. J Arthroplasty 2007;22(6 Suppl 2):140–4.

5. Matta JM, Shahrdar C, Ferguson T. Single-incision anterior approach for total hip arthroplasty on an orthopaedic table. Clin Orthop Relat Res 2005;441:115–24.

6. Siguier T, Siguier M, Brumpt B. Mini-incision anterior approach does not increase dislocation rate: a study of 1037 total hip replacements. Clin Orthop Relat Res 2004;426:164–73.

7. Meneghini RM, Pagnano MW, Trousdale RT, et al. Muscle damage during MIS total hip arthroplasty: Smith-Petersen versus posterior approach. Clin Orthop Relat Res 2006;453:293–8.

8. Barber TC, Roger DJ, Goodman SB, et al. Early outcome of total hip arthroplasty using the direct lateral vs the posterior surgical approach. Orthopedics 1996;19(10):873–5.

9. Carlson DC, Robinson HJ Jr. Surgical approaches for primary total hip arthroplasty. A prospective comparison of the Marcy modification of the Gibson and Watson-Jones approaches. Clin Orthop Relat Res 1987;222:161–6.

10. Horwitz BR, Rockowitz NL, Goll SR, et al. A prospective randomized comparison of two surgical approaches to total hip arthroplasty. Clin Orthop Relat Res 1993;291:154–63.

11. Nakata K, Nishikawa M, Yamamoto K, et al. A clinical comparative study of the direct anterior with mini-posterior approach. Two consecutive series. J Arthroplasty 2008, epub ahead of print.

12. Ward SR, Jones RE, Long WT, et al. Functional recovery of muscles after minimally invasive total hip arthroplasty. Instr Course Lect 2008;57:249–54.

13. Maffiuletti NA, Gorelick M, Kramers-de Quervain I, et al. Concurrent validity and intrasession reliability of the IDEEA accelerometry system for the quantification of spatiotemporal gait parameters. Gait Posture 2008;27(1):160–3.

14. Judet J, Judet R. The use of an artificial femoral head for arthroplasty of the hip joint. J Bone Joint Surg Br 1950;32-B(2):166–73.

15. Smith-Petersen MN. Approach to and exposure of the hip joint for mold arthroplasty. J Bone Joint Surg Am 1949;31A(1):40–6.

16. Trudelle-Jackson E, Smith SS. Effects of a late-phase exercise program after total hip arthroplasty: a randomized controlled trial. Arch Phys Med Rehabil 2004;85(7):1056–62.

17. Brooker AF, Bowerman JW, Robinson RA, et al. Ectopic ossification following total hip replacement. Incidence and a method of classification. J Bone Joint Surg Am 1973;55(8):1629–32.

18. Stucki G, Meier D, Stucki S, et al. Evaluation of a German version of WOMAC (Western Ontario and McMaster Universities) Arthrosis Index. Z Rheumatol 1996;55(1):40–9.

19. Ware JE, Kosinski M, Keller SD. SF-12: how to score the SF-12 physical and mental component health summary scales. Second edition. Boston: The Health Institute, New England Medical Center; 1995.

20. Gandek B, Ware JE, Aaronson NK, et al. Cross-validation of item selection and scoring for the SF-12 Health Survey in nine countries: results from the IQOLA Project. International Quality of Life Assessment. J Clin Epidemiol 1998;51:1171–8.

21. Bilney B, Morris M, Webster K. Concurrent related validity of the GAITRite walkway system for quantification of the spatial and temporal parameters of gait. Gait Posture 2003;17(1):68–74.

22. Menz HB, Latt MD, Tiedemann A, et al. Reliability of the GAITRite walkway system for the quantification of temporo-spatial parameters of gait in young and older people. Gait Posture 2004;20(1):20–5.

23. Berman AT, Zarro VJ, Bosacco SJ, et al. Quantitative gait analysis after unilateral or bilateral total knee replacement. J Bone Joint Surg Am 1987;69(9): 1340–5.

24. Simon SR, Trieshmann HW, Burdett RG, et al. Quantitative gait analysis after total knee arthroplasty for monarticular degenerative arthritis. J Bone Joint Surg Am 1983;65(5):605–13.

25. Cohen J. Statistical power analysis for the behavioral sciences. 2nd edition. Hillsdale (NJ): Lawrence Earlbaum Associates; 1988.

26. Perry J. Gait analysis: normal and pathological function. New York: McGraw Hill, Inc.; 1992.

27. Lyons K, Perry J, Gronley JK, et al. Timing and relative intensity of hip extensor and abductor muscle action during level and stair ambulation: an EMG study. Phys Ther 1983;63:1597–605.

28. Andriacchi TP, Galante JO, Fermier RW. The influence of total knee-replacement design on walking and stair-climbing. J Bone Joint Surg Am 1982; 64(9):1328–35.

29. Webster KE, Wittwer JE, Feller JA. Quantitative gait analysis after medial unicompartmental knee arthroplasty for osteoarthritis. J Arthroplasty 2003;18(6): 751–9.

30. Andriacchi TP, Ogle JA, Galante JO. Walking speed as a basis for normal and abnormal gait measurements. J Biomech 1977;10:261–8.

31. Mattsson E, Olsson E, Brostrom LA. Assessment of walking before and after unicompartmental knee arthroplasty. A comparison of different methods. Scand J Rehabil Med 1990;22(1):45–50.

32. Bennett D, Ogonda L, Elliott D, et al. Comparison of gait kinematics in patients receiving minimally invasive and traditional hip replacement surgery: a prospective blinded study. Gait Posture 2006;23: 374–82.

33. Madsen MS, Ritter MA, Morris HH, et al. The effect of total hip arthroplasty surgical approach on gait. J Orthop Res 2004;22:44–50.

34. Meneghini RM, Smits SA, Swinford RR, et al. A randomized, prospective study of 3 minimally invasive surgical approaches in total hip arthroplasty. J Arthroplasty 2008;23(6):68–73.

35. Mont MA, Seyler TM, Ragland PS, et al. Gait analysis of patients with resurfacing hip arthroplasty compared with hip ostheoarthritis and standard total hip arthroplasty. J Arthroplasty 2007;22(1): 100–8.

36. Dorr L, Maheshwari AV, Long WT, et al. Early pain relief and function after posterior minimally invasive and conventional total hip arthroplasty. J Bone Joint Surg Am 2007;89:1153–60.

37. Mardones R, Pagnano MW, Nemanich JP, et al. The Frank Stinchfield Award: muscle damage after total hip arthroplasty done with the two-incision and mini-posterior techniques. Clin Orthop Relat Res 2005;441:63–7.

Blood Management for Hip Reconstruction Surgery

Alan Lane, MB, FCARCSI*, Edward T. Crosby, MD, FRCPC

KEYWORDS

• Blood conservation • Transfusion • Hip reconstruction

Red cell transfusion is a common component of care in hip reconstruction surgery. Efforts to reduce the incidence and volume of transfusion have been reinforced recently for a number of reasons. First, blood transfusion is associated with both increased morbidity and postoperative length of stay. Second, blood components are a limited health care resource; their administration should be restricted to scenarios whereby they confer a benefit on the recipient. Finally, despite the enormous and largely successful efforts made to enhance blood safety in the North American blood systems, many patients remain skeptical about transfusion safety and would prefer to avoid allogeneic transfusion.[1] In the following article, we review the likelihood of transfusion events in reconstruction surgery and the risks and benefits of transfusion, and evolve strategies to reduce patient exposure to allogeneic blood perioperatively.

RISKS OF RED BLOOD CELL TRANSFUSION

Infectious disease testing has dramatically improved the safety of blood for transfusion in the North America, especially since the introduction of nucleic acid amplification testing.[2] The current estimated residual risk of HIV and hepatitis C virus transmission through blood transfusion is estimated to be approximately one case in 2 million transfusion events. Hepatitis B virus risk remains at one case in 200,000–500,000

transfusion events. Although there were early cases of transfusion-transmitted West Nile virus, none have been reported since the test sensitivity was increased in epidemic areas. Serious noninfectious complications from blood component transfusion are now more likely to occur than viral disease transmission.[3] These reactions may result from immunologic incompatibility between donor and host, bacterial contamination of the blood product administered, or from the volume of product transfused to patients who have limited cardiovascular reserve. An increased incidence of postoperative infectious complications also occurs in transfusion recipients and may result from modulation of the immune system function in the recipient. The use of universal leukodepletion at the time of donor unit collection may reduce such immunomodulation and the subsequent infectious sequelae.

PREDICTING THE LIKELIHOOD OF RED CELL TRANSFUSION DURING HIP RECONSTRUCTION

The likelihood of a patient receiving a transfusion after hip surgery has been assessed by a number of investigators; the major determinants are the initial hemoglobin concentration ([Hb_i]) and the perioperative blood loss. In a review of 9482 subjects who underwent total hip or knee arthroplasty, the lower the [Hb_i], the more probable the transfusion of allogeneic blood.[4] Of the 3020 subjects who had an [Hb_i] greater than 10 g/dL^{-1}

Department of Anesthesiology, The Ottawa Hospital, General Campus, 501 Smyth Road, Ottawa, ON K1H 8L6, Canada
* Corresponding author.
E-mail address: alantlane@yahoo.co.uk (A. Lane).

Orthop Clin N Am 40 (2009) 417–425
doi:10.1016/j.ocl.2009.02.003

but less than or equal to 13 g/dL^{-1}, 864 (29%) required a transfusion compared with 267 (8%) of 3374 subjects who had [Hb$_i$] greater than 14 g/dL^{-1}. In addition to an [Hb$_i$] of 12 g/dL^{-1} or less, positive associations exist between transfusion risk and age over 65 years, female sex, weight 60 kg or less, ASA classification greater than II, and revision surgery.[5] The use of acetylsalicylic acid has also been reported to increase the risk of red cell transfusions after total hip arthroplasty.[6]

Blood loss can be considerable during arthroplasty surgery and is often underestimated because the losses may not be obvious or easily measurable.[7] In a large multicenter analysis of blood management in subjects undergoing elective hip arthroplasty, the mean *estimated* blood loss for total hip arthroplasty was 750 mLs, whereas the actual *measured* loss was 1944 mLs. The blood loss that can be safely tolerated by a patient is directly related not only to the [Hb$_i$] but also to the patient's blood volume. Blood volume may be estimated in adults as being between 65–75 mL/kg^{-1}. The blood volume that a patient may lose and yet still maintain their [Hb] at a safe level has been termed the *safe allowable blood loss*. The higher the safe allowable blood loss that the patient will tolerate, the lower is the risk that they will require perioperative transfusion. In subjects undergoing primary or revision total hip replacement, those who had a safe allowable blood loss of 850 mLs or less were more likely to receive a postoperative transfusion than those who had a safe allowable loss greater than 850 mLs.[8] Although complicated formulae do exist to calculate allowable blood loss, there is a reasonable correlation between the measure of the percentage of estimated blood volume lost and the reduction in [Hb]. That is, if the blood lost perioperatively represents about 25% of the estimated blood volume, one can expect that the resulting [Hb] will be reduced in similar proportion from baseline levels.

Table 1
Risk factors for transfusion with hip reconstruction
Initial Hb level < 12 g-dl^{-1}
Weight < 60 kg
Age > 65 years
Major revision or pelvic surgery
Female sex
ASA classification > II
Presence of major cardiovascular disease

ANEMIA — INCIDENCE AND CONSEQUENCES

Anemia is very common in patients hospitalized for surgical interventions and is associated with increased morbidity and mortality and an increased length of hospital stay.[9] Conversely, a higher [Hb$_i$] in patients presenting with hip fracture is associated with shorter lengths of hospital stay and lower odds of readmission or death.[10] It is not clear whether the effects on outcome are caused by the anemia per se or by an association with other risk factors frequently prevalent in anemic patients. Variances from normal hematocrits (HCT) are associated with poor postoperative outcomes whether the HCT was lower or higher than normal values.[11] Even mild degrees of anemia or polycythemia are associated with an increased 30-day mortality and cardiac events in elderly patients undergoing major noncardiac surgery, suggesting that the comorbidity influencing the [Hb] may be as or even more relevant to outcome than the measured [Hb].

The extent of comorbidities may also amplify the adverse effects of a low [Hb] which in turn may have been a surrogate marker for severe underlying diseases. For example, anemia is linked as an independent risk factor for increased mortality, morbidity, increased length of hospital stay, and increased mortality in patients who have congestive heart failure or left ventricular dysfunction.[12] However, despite the association of anemia with cardiovascular morbidity and mortality, the presence of cardiac risk factors have not predicted the occurrence of silent myocardial ischemia perioperatively in patients undergoing major lower limb joint replacement surgery.[13] Nor has a restrictive (8 g/dL^{-1}) transfusion trigger resulted in an increased incidence of silent ischemia when compared with a more liberal (10 g/dL^{-1}) trigger in patients having elective hip and knee replacement surgery.[14] It may be that concurrent anemia amplifies the severity of illness when cardiac decompensation has occurred but does not usually cause it alone, even in at-risk patients who have a stable cardiovascular condition.

The lowest safe level of anemia was assessed by Carson and colleagues[15] in a retrospective cohort study of subjects over the age of 18 years who declined red cell transfusions for religious reasons. Of the 2083 subjects reviewed, 300 had postoperative [Hb] of 8 g/dL^{-1} or less. In subjects who had postoperative [Hb] of 7.1 to 8 g/dL^{-1}, none died and 9.4% had a morbid event. In subjects who had [Hb] of 4.1 to 5 g/dL^{-1}, 34.4% died and 57.7% had a morbid event. The odds of death in subjects who had a postoperative [Hb] of 8 g/dL^{-1} or less increased 2.5 times for each g/dL^{-1} decrease in [Hb].

THE IMPACT OF ANEMIA ON FUNCTIONAL STATUS AND EFFICIENCY OF REHABILITATION

A higher postoperative [Hb] may improve functional recovery after hip fracture repair and facilitate postoperative rehabilitation.[16] The predicted distance walked at discharge in patients undergoing hip fracture repair is increased in patients who have higher [Hb]; after adjustment for other factors associated with ability to walk, higher [Hb] were independently associated with walking greater distances. A higher baseline [Hb] was also associated with a significantly shorter length of stay and improved patient function during rehabilitation after primary total knee arthroplasty.[17] Although, there is some evidence for improved efficiency of rehabilitation in association with higher [Hb] after hip fracture repair, functional scores after hip arthroplasty do not correlate with postoperative [Hb].[18] Similarly, though there are limited data that suggest that rehabilitation is more efficient in patients who have higher [Hb], the majority of rehabilitation physicians surveyed would transfuse patients who have a HCT below 25, suggesting that there is a consensus in clinical opinion that a low [Hb] has a negative impact on the efficiency of rehabilitation.[19]

IMPACT OF A GUIDANCE PROTOCOL ON TRANSFUSION PRACTICES IN ORTHOPEDIC SURGERY

The use of institutional protocols or care pathways increases the use of alternatives to allogeneic transfusion and decreases the incidence of blood transfusion after joint arthroplasty. A simple, one-page flowchart that summarizes graphically the perioperative decision pathways for anemic patients, placed in the charts of all patients undergoing total joint replacement and given out to medical staff, resulted in a decrease in the proportion of patients receiving blood transfusion from 35% to 19.8%.[20] Similarly, the application of a transfusion algorithm after primary knee and hip arthroplasty resulted in a 56% reduction in transfusions (both autologous and allogeneic), a 50% reduction in the number of wasted autologous units, and a 50% reduction in hospital costs related to transfusion.[21] The use of a preoperative blood conservation algorithm (BCA) in patients having total hip arthroplasty reduced the allogeneic transfusion rate to 16.5% compared with 26.1% for those assigned to usual care (UC), an absolute risk reduction of 9.6%.[22] For patients who had a preoperative [Hb] of 10.1–13.0 g/dL^{-1}, the allogeneic transfusion rate was 24.6% in the BCA arm versus 47.6% in the UC arm, an absolute risk reduction of 23%.

FACTORS THAT INFLUENCE BLOOD LOSS

There are a number of factors in addition to surgical techniques and duration of surgery that may influence intraoperative blood losses during hip arthroplasty surgery. The use of antiplatelet drugs, anticoagulants, and nonsteroidal anti-inflammatory drugs (NSAIDs) should be identified preoperatively, allowing adequate time for discontinuation before surgery. Although the use of NSAIDs has been associated with increased perioperative blood loss, discontinuing them preoperatively can result in a hyperalgesic pain state.[23] The use of celecoxib perioperatively maintains the benefit of COX 2 inhibition without effecting platelet function and it may be substituted for other NSAIDs in patients without contraindications.

Anesthesia techniques can also influence blood loss. The use of spinal anesthesia for hip arthroplasty surgery results in a reduction in the risk of blood transfusion.[24] Beyond the reduction in risk of blood transfusion, neuraxial blockade with spinal and epidural anesthesia reduces postoperative morbidity and mortality, including the incidence of deep vein thrombosis, pulmonary embolism, respiratory depression, pneumonia, and myocardial infarction.[25] In cases of hypotensive anesthesia, whereby the mean arterial pressure is decreased from 60 mm to 50 mm Hg with the use of epidural anesthesia, also reduces mean intraoperative blood loss. However, the decreases are typically modest and the clinical relevance of such decreases in reducing the requirement for transfusion is questioned. In addition, invasive monitoring is required, adding to the complexity of this technique.[26]

An often ignored risk factor for perioperative blood loss is patient hypothermia. Perioperative hypothermia reduces platelet function and impairs the function of the enzymes of the coagulation cascade. Even mild hypothermia ($\leq 1°$ C) significantly increases blood loss and the relative risk of transfusion. Maintaining perioperative normothermia reduces blood loss and transfusion requirements by clinically important amounts.[27]

ALTERNATIVES TO ALLOGENEIC TRANSFUSION

The likelihood that a patient will receive an allogeneic transfusion after joint arthroplasty is determined largely by patient weight, comorbidities, blood volume, [Hb$_i$] and surgical blood losses. Surgical blood losses will vary but are influenced by both the operator and the duration of surgery;

total perioperative losses of 1–1.5 L and a decrease in [Hb] of 3–4.5 g/dL^{-1} are typical in our experience. There are some patients who would be predicted to be at low risk for blood transfusion; the intensity of transfusion avoidance strategies applied to the care of the individual patient should be in proportion to the likelihood that an individual patient will require a blood transfusion. However, an organized approach to transfusion at the institutional level seems to result in more appropriate transfusion regimes, fewer inappropriate transfusions, and less wasted blood in the patient population. Most patients who weigh more than 60 kg and have a preoperative [Hb] greater than 14 g/dL^{-1} are at relatively low risk (<10%) for perioperative transfusion and should probably be allowed to proceed to reconstructive surgery without any advance blood avoidance strategies in place.[4] A blood conservation strategy should be considered for patients who have [Hb$_i$]

greater than 10 g/dL^{-1} and less than 14 g/dL^{-1} (**Fig. 1**). If the [Hb$_i$] is less than 10 g/dL^{-1}, consideration should be given to delaying surgery to investigate the low [Hb] and institute strategies to correct the anemia.

STRATEGIES AND INTERVENTIONS TO REDUCE ALLOGENEIC TRANSFUSION
Autologous Predonation

Autologous predonation (APD) can be considered for patients presenting for hip reconstruction surgery and considered likely to require transfusion (**Table 1**).

However, drawing blood from patients at low risk for perioperative transfusion increases unit wastage and care costs and provides little benefit to most patients. Autologous donation will reduce [Hb] in all patients and most will not recover their [Hb] to baseline levels in the preoperative period

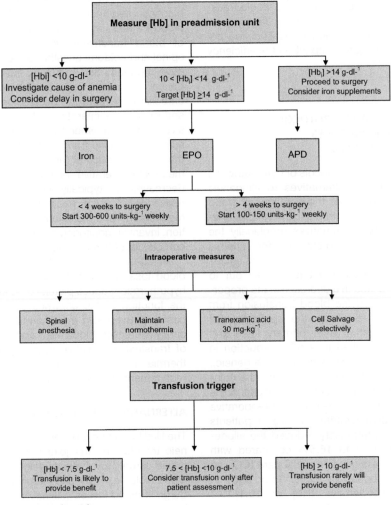

Fig. 1. Blood conservation algorithm.

in the absence of EPO treatment; many at low risk for transfusion will thus be shifted into a higher risk group as a result of the phlebotomy.[28] As the goal of APD is to reduce allogeneic exposure for patients considered to be more likely to receive transfusion, it should be supported with EPO and iron therapy in the preoperative period to allow for recovery to baseline [Hb] before surgery.

Erythropoietin

The administration of preoperative EPO therapy has been approved for both patients donating autologous blood before surgery and those who will not donate blood; analysis of randomized trials affirm the effectiveness of this strategy in reducing the risk for perioperative transfusion in patients at higher risk.[29] It should be considered for patients presenting for hip reconstruction who are deemed to be at higher risk for transfusion whether they intend to participate in autologous programs or not. Although serial doses as low as 60 units/kg^{-1} will stimulate modest but sustained increases in erythropoiesis, doses of less than 100 units/kg^{-1} are not effective in facilitating autologous donation and cannot be recommended.[30] If time permits, it is reasonable to begin EPO therapy with doses of 100–150 units/kg^{-1}; if an inadequate response is seen with this dosing, larger doses (300–600 units/kg^{-1}) should then be considered. If the interval to surgery is shorter, consideration should be given to the use of larger doses (300–600 units/kg^{-1}) from the outset. EPO therapy should be started at least 2 weeks before surgery; efficacy will be enhanced with therapy of longer duration and is diminished or absent with therapy of shorter duration. The HCT begins to rise within several days of EPO administration; one unit of blood is produced per week of treatment. Weekly doses of EPO are as effective as daily administration and less expensive, and subcutaneous administration is convenient and effective. All patients should be administered supplemental iron during EPO therapy and oral iron (ferrous sulfate 325 mg three times a day) is usually adequate.

Although there is concern is about the development of thrombotic complications associated with the higher HCT resulting from EPO therapy, analysis of data from four randomized studies involving 869 subjects undergoing major, elective orthopedic surgery reported that the incidence of thrombotic/vascular events was similar between subjects treated with EPO and those receiving placebo (7.4% versus 8.0%, respectively).[31] In this analysis, age, cardiac history, hypertension, and cardiac medications, but not EPO, were determined to be risk factors for thrombotic/vascular events. Similarly, an analysis of randomized trials also reported that there is no convincing evidence that EPO increased the frequency of thrombotic complications, but noted that some studies reviewed found an excess of events in EPO-treated subjects.[32]

Iron Supplementation Therapy

Approximately 20% of patients who present for joint reconstructive surgery have coexisting anemia. While the majority of these patients will have an anemia reflective of chronic disease, some (20%) will have an anemia responsive to iron therapy.[33] Preoperative oral iron supplementation reduces transfusion requirements in orthopedic surgery. While oral administration is the usual route, intravenous iron is an alternative particularly in patients who are intolerant of oral iron and when time to surgery is short. Intravenous iron can also improve the response to EPO, allowing for a reduction in dose requirements.[34]

Pharmacologic Approaches to Reduce Bleeding and Transfusion

Pharmacologic agents used to reduce perioperative blood loss include the antifibrinolytic drugs aprotinin, tranexamic acid (TXA), and epsilon aminocaproic acid (EACA). Both aprotinin and TXA have been demonstrated to reduce surgical blood loss and allogeneic red blood cell transfusion.[35] In the case of EACA, the evidence of its clinical benefit is equivocal, and limited by the small number of trials involving this drug. Aprotinin appears to be the most effective transfusion-sparing agent for cardiac surgery but an advantage over TXA has not been reported in orthopedic surgery. However, recent publications that reported an increased incidence of renal failure, myocardial infarction, and all-cause mortality with the use of aprotinin in cardiac surgery led to its withdrawal from the market in November 2007.[36]

A recent meta-analysis comprising 1084 subjects from 20 studies involving primary hip and knee arthroplasty reported that treatment with TXA but not EACA led to a reduction in the proportion of primary hip arthroplasty patients requiring at least one unit of allogeneic red cell transfusion, given according to a transfusion protocol.[37] The results also suggested improved efficacy with more than a single dose of TXA, with either repeated boluses or a continuous infusion being superior to a single dose. Although this meta-analysis did not detect an excess risk of thromboembolic events with the use of TXA, no definite conclusion could be drawn on these adverse risks due to the small sample sizes of the trials and the low baseline incidences of serious adverse events. The use of TXA in patients who have increased risk of thrombotic events needs to be individually reviewed.

Published studies have used a variety of dosing regimes for TXA and the optimal dosing schedule for perioperative TXA remains uncertain. Our practice has been to administer a total dose of about 30 mg/kg^{-1}, given in divided doses, with the first dose given pre-incision and the second dose either at the end of surgery or in the postoperative care unit.

Acute Normovolemic Hemodilution

Guidelines for the use of acute normovolemic hemodilution (ANH) suggest its consideration if the potential surgical blood loss is expected to exceed 20% of the patient's blood volume and the [Hb$_i$] is greater than 10 g/dL^{-1} in the absence of coronary artery disease.[38] The value of AHN depends on the degree of hemodilution achieved and mathematical modeling demonstrates that extreme hemodilution with target HCT of 20% followed by substantial blood loss would be required before the red cell volume saved by hemodilution becomes clinically significant.[39] A recent meta-analysis reviewed 42 trials comparing ANH with usual care or to another blood conservation technique. While demonstrating no reduction in the proportion of patients exposed to allogeneic blood, those in the ANH group who were actually transfused received 1–2 units less.[40] A study of ANH in subjects undergoing elective primary and revision hip surgery with ANH to a target [Hb] level of 11 g/dL^{-1} reported no reduction in allogeneic blood transfusion in the ANH group. There was, however, a threefold reduction in infectious complications compared with standard transfusion.[41] The benefits of ANH appear modest and can be considered equivalent to APD.[42]

Intraoperative Cell Salvage

Cell salvage devices are beneficial in surgical procedures involving substantial blood loss and can provide the equivalent of 10 units of autologous blood per hour in patients who have massive bleeding. Infection, malignancy, and contaminants such as amniotic fluid, ascites, and hydrogen peroxide solutions are the main contraindications to the use of intraoperative cell salvage. The equivalent of at least two units of blood needs to be routinely recovered in order for this method to be cost effective. A recent study on cell salvage in revision hip surgery demonstrated a reduction in allogeneic red cell transfusion requirements from a median of six units to two units with intraoperative cell salvage.[43] A similar study reviewing intraoperative cell salvage combined with tranexamic acid in revision hip surgery demonstrated a reduction in allogeneic blood usage of 62.5% in the treatment group compared with the control group.[44] In our experience, the routine use of cell salvage for primary hip replacement is not indicated because intraoperative collection is often inconsequential. However, its use should be considered in surgeries with predicted significant blood losses particularly if other risk factors for transfusion are present (see above), in patients who have significant blood-matching issues and in patients resistant to the administration of allogeneic blood for religious or other reasons.

Recommendations

Minimizing perioperative blood transfusion during the course of hip reconstruction may involve the application of several blood conservation techniques (**Table 2**). Ideally, patients should be seen sufficiently well in advance of surgery to allow adequate time to minimize transfusion risk by maximizing their safe allowable blood loss. Patients who have [Hb$_i$] less than 10 g/dL^{-1} should have the cause of their anemia investigated; it may be necessary to defer surgery until the issue is resolved. Patients of at least average size and stature and who have a [Hb$_i$] greater than 14 g/dL^{-1} will not likely require transfusion in most cases and treatment with oral iron should be provided at the time they are scheduled for surgery.

Patients who have [Hb$_i$] between 10 g/dL^{-1} and 14 g/dL^{-1} are most likely to benefit from interventions to raise their preoperative [Hb]. Iron supplementation, together with folate and vitamin B12 when appropriate, are low-cost interventions that should be routinely implemented. EPO is more costly but is an effective way to increase [Hb]. Provided that there is sufficient time to assess response and adjust dosing, patients in higher risk groups can commence EPO therapy at 100–150 units/kg^{-1} weekly, targeting a final preoperative [Hb] of 14 g/dL^{-1} or greater. If time is short, therapy should commence with doses of 300–600 units/kg^{-1} weekly.

APD is recommended for the following circumstances: (1) for patients who have particular concerns regarding allogeneic blood transfusion, (2) if the availability or suitability of appropriate allogeneic blood is an issue, or (3) if larger losses are anticipated as in the case of revision surgery or bilateral reconstruction. Adequate time must

Table 2
Summary of blood conservation techniques for hip reconstruction surgery.

Intervention	Advantage	Disadvantage
EPO	Effective means of raising preoperative [Hb].	Costly. Needs to commence at least 2 weeks preoperatively. Requires injection.
Autologous predonation	Useful if allogeneic blood transfusion problematic. Suitable for cases with larger anticipated blood losses.	Interval required for recovery of [Hb] to baseline. Optimally requires EPO and iron support.
Acute normovolemic hemodilution	Can be instituted on day of surgery. Provides whole blood for retransfusion. Useful if difficulty obtaining allogeneic blood.	Practical issues with venesection. Contraindicated in patients with significant cardiac or respiratory disease.
Cell salvage	Easy to implement. Provides immediate suitable blood. Useful in major revision surgery.	Costly. Low yields in primary arthroplasty. Technical set-up of circuit.
Tranexamic acid	Suitable in patients at low risk of thromboembolic events. Ease of administration.	Contraindicated in patients at increased risk of thromboembolic events.

be allowed for recovery of baseline [Hb] and APD should be supported with EPO and iron administration.

Intraoperatively, the use of spinal anesthesia together with aggressive maintenance of normothermia is recommended. Tranexamic acid, in a total dose of 30 mg/kg^{-1}, given in two divided doses, the first pre-incision and the second within 2–3 hours, is recommended in patients who are not at increased risk of thromboembolic events.

It is our opinion that the use of either ANH or cell salvage is not indicated for primary hip arthroplasty but that it should be considered for surgeries with greater anticipated blood losses (>1500 mL) and again if there are blood incompatibility issues or a refusal to accept allogeneic transfusion. Typically, the collection and processing apparatus of the cell salvage machine can be set up separately; if sufficient volumes of blood are collected, the processing system may then be deployed.

The decision to transfuse allogeneic red cells should be made after a review of a patient's age, medical condition, and cardiovascular reserve, ongoing blood losses, tolerance of anemia and the ability to recover [Hb]. Most patients who have [Hb] below 7.5 g/dL^{-1} will likely require transfusion even if hemodynamically stable. Patients who have [Hb] between 7.5 g/dL^{-1} and 10 g/dL^{-1} will require individual assessment of the

above factors; many will prove relatively intolerant of [Hb] of 8 g/dL^{-1} or less. Older, frail patients who have cardiovascular disease will likely benefit from having [Hb] maintained somewhat higher in the range identified (between 9–10 g/dL^{-1}). Patients who have [Hb] of 10 g/dL^{-1} or greater will rarely require or benefit from transfusion.

SUMMARY

Hip reconstruction surgery is suitable for the application of blood conservation techniques. An organized, systematic approach to this patient group, together with an incremental patient-focused strategy can maximize the benefits offered by these techniques. Cost and resource implications can be balanced by reduced transfusion requirements and patient morbidity.

REFERENCES

1. Finucane ML, Slovic P, Mertz CK. Public perception of the risk of blood transfusion. Transfusion 2000;40: 1017–22.
2. Stramer SL. Current risks of transfusion transmitted agents. Arch Pathol Lab Med 2007;131:702–7.
3. Eder AF, Chambers LA. Noninfectious complications of a blood transfusion. Arch Pathol Lab Med 2007; 131:708–18.

4. Bierbaum BE, Callaghan JJ, Galante JO, et al. An analysis of blood management in patients having a total hip or knee arthroplasty. J Bone Joint Surg Am 1999;81:2–10.

5. Rashiq S, Shah M, Chow AK, et al. Predicting allogeneic blood transfusion use in total joint arthroplasty. Anesth Analg 2004;99:1239–44.

6. Nuttal GA, Santrach PJ, Oliver WC Jr, et al. The predictors of red cell transfusions in total hip arthroplasties. Transfusion 1996;36:144–9.

7. Rosencher N, Kerkkamp HE, Macheras G, et al. The Orthopedic Surgery Transfusion Hemoglobin European Overview (OSTHEO) study: lead management in elective knee and hip arthroplasty in Europe. Transfusion 2003;43:459–69.

8. Nelson CL, Stewart JG. Primary and revision total hip replacement in patients who are Jehovah's Witnesses. Clin Orthop 1999;369:251–61.

9. Dunne JR, Malone D, Tracy JK, et al. Perioperative anemia: an independent risk factor for infection, mortality, and resource utilization in surgery. J Surg Res 2002;102:237–44.

10. Halm EA, Wang JJ, Boockvar K, et al. The effect of perioperative anemia on clinical and functional outcomes in patients with hip fracture. J Orthop Trauma 2004;18:369–74.

11. Wu WC, Schifftner TL, Henderson WG, et al. Preoperative hematocrit levels and postoperative outcomes in older patients undergoing noncardiac surgery. JAMA 2007;297:2481–8.

12. Spence RK. Medical and economic impact of anemia in hospitalized patients. Am J Health Syst Pharm 2007;64:S3–10.

13. French GW, Lam WH, Rashid Z, et al. Perioperative silent myocardial ischemia in patients undergoing lower limb joint replacement surgery: an indicator of postoperative morbidity or mortality? Anaesthesia 1999;54:235–40.

14. Grover M, Talwalkar S, Casbard A, et al. Silent myocardial ischaemia and haemoglobin concentration: a randomized controlled trial of transfusion strategy in lower limb of arthroplasty. Vox Sang 2006;90:105–12.

15. Carson JL, Noveck H, Berlin JA, et al. Mortality and morbidity in patients with very low postoperative hemoglobin levels who declined blood transfusion. Transfusion 2002;42:812–8.

16. Lawrence VA, Silverstein JH, Cornell JE, et al. Higher hemoglobin level is associated with better early functional recovery after hip fracture repair. Transfusion 2003;43:1717–22.

17. Diamond PT, Conaway MR, Mody SH, et al. Influence of hemoglobin levels on inpatient rehabilitation outcomes after total knee arthroplasty. J Arthroplasty 2006;21:636–41.

18. Wallis JP, Wells AW, Whitehead S, et al. Recovery from postoperative anemia. Transfus Med 2005;15: 413–8.

19. Diamond PT, Julian DM. Practice trends in the management of low hematocrit in the acute rehabilitation setting. Am J Phys Med Rehabil 2001;8(11): 816–20.

20. Muller U, Exadaktylos A, Roeder C, et al. Effect of a flowchart on use of blood transfusions in primary total hip and knee replacement: prospective before and after study. Br Med J 2004;328:934–8.

21. Marinez V, Monsaingeon-Lion A, Cherif K, et al. Transfusion strategy for primary knee and hip arthroplasty: impact of an algorithm to lower transfusion rates and hospital costs. Br J Anaesth 2007;99:794–800.

22. Wong CJ, Vandervoort MK, Vandervoort SL, et al. A cluster randomized controlled trial of a blood conservation algorithm in patients undergoing total hip joint arthroplasty. Transfusion 2007;47: 832–41.

23. Robinson CM, Christie J, Malcolm-Smith N. Non steroidal anti inflammatory drugs, perioperative blood loss, transfusion requirements in elective hip surgery. J Arthroplasty 1993;8:607–10.

24. Rashiq S, Finegan B. The effect of spinal anesthesia on blood transfusion rate in total joint arthroplasty. Can J Surg 2006;49(6):391–6.

25. Rodgers A, Walker N, Shug S, et al. Reduction of postoperative mortality and morbidity with epidural and spinal anaesthesia: results from overview of randomized trials. BMJ 2000;321(7275): 1493.

26. Sharrock NE, Salvati EA. Hypotensive epidural anesthesia for total hip arthroplasty. Acta Orthop Scand 1996;67:17–25.

27. Rajagopalan S, Mascha E, Na J, et al. The effects of mild perioperative hypothermia on blood loss and transfusion requirements. Anesthesiology 2008; 108:71–7.

28. Cushner FD, Hawes T, Kessler D, et al. Orthopaedic-induced anemia; the fallacy of autologous donation programs. Clin Orthop Rel Res 2005;431:145–9.

29. Laupacis A, Fergusson D. Erythropoietin to minimize perioperative blood transfusion: a systematic review of randomized trials. The International Study of Perioperative Transfusion (ISPOT) Investigators. Transfus Med 1998;8:309–17.

30. Sans T, Joven J, Vilella E, et al. Pharmacokinetics of several subcutaneous doses of erythropoietin: implications for blood transfusion. Clin Exp Pharmacol Physiol 2000;27:179–84.

31. de Andrade JR, Frei D, Guilfoyle M. Integrated analysis of thrombotic/vascular event occurrence in epoetin alfa-treated patients undergoing major, elective orthopedic surgery. Orthopedics 1999; 22(1 Suppl):S113–8.

32. Canadian Orthopaedic Perioperative Erythropoietin Study Group. Effectiveness of perioperative recombinant human erythropoietin in elective hip replacement. Lancet 1993;341:1227–32.

33. Saleh E, McClelland DB, Hay A, et al. Prevalence of anaemia before major joint arthroplasty and the potential impact of preoperative investigation and correction on perioperative blood transfusions. Br J Anaesth 2007;99(6):801–7.

34. Beris P, Munoz M, Garcia-Erce JA, et al. Perioperative anaemia management: consensus statement on the role of intravenous iron. Br J Anaesth 2008; 100(5):599–604.

35. Henry DA, Carless PA, Moxey AJ, et al. Antifibrinolytic use for minimising perioperative allogeneic blood transfusion. Cochrane Database Syst Rev 2007;4:CD001886.

36. Levy JH. Pharmacological methods to reduce perioperative bleeding. Transfusion 2008;48:31S–8S.

37. Zuffery P, Marquiol F, Laporte S, et al. Do antifibrinolytics reduce allogeneic blood transfusion in orthopedic surgery? Anesthesiology 2006;105: 1034–46.

38. Napier JA, Bruce M, Chapman J, et al. Guidelines for autologous transfusion. II. Perioperative haemodilution and cell salvage. Br J Anaesth 1997;78: 768–71.

39. Brecher ME, Rosenfield M. Mathematical and computer modeling of acute normovolemic hemodilution. Transfusion 1994;34:176–9.

40. Segal J, Blasco-Colmenares E, Norris E, et al. Preoperative acute normovolemic hemodilution; a meta-analysis. Transfusion 2004;44(5):1097–103.

41. Bennet J, Haynes S, Torella F, et al. Acute normovolemic hemodilution in moderate blood loss surgery: a randomized controlled trial. Transfusion 2006;46: 1097–103.

42. Goodnough L, Despotis G, Merkel K, et al. A randomized trial comparing acute normovolemic hemodilution and preoperative autologous blood donation in total hip arthroplasty. Transfusion 2000; 40:1054–7.

43. Bridgens JP, Evans CR, Dobson PM, et al. Intraoperative red blood cell salvage in revision hip surgery. A case matched study. J Bone Joint Surg Am 2007;89(2):270–5.

44. Philips SJ, Chavan R, Porter ML, et al. Does salvage and tranexamic acid reduce the need for blood transfusion in revision hip surgery? J Bone Joint Surg Br 2006;88-B:1141–2.

Overview of Current Venous Thromboembolism Protocols in Hip Reconstruction

Alejandro Lazo-Langner, MD, MSc[a,b,c],
Marc A. Rodger, MD, MSc, FRCPC[d,e,f,g],*

KEYWORDS

- Total hip arthroplasty • Prophylaxis • Anticoagulants
- Venous thrombosis • Pulmonary embolism

OVERVIEW OF VENOUS THROMBOEMBOLIC DISEASE

Venous thromboembolic disease, or venous thromboembolism (VTE), is a serious and frequent complication of orthopedic surgery. It comprises two clinical entities which, from a treatment and etiologic perspective, are considered the same condition: (1) deep vein thrombosis (DVT), when a thrombus develops in a deep vein; and (2) pulmonary embolism (PE), when the thrombus detaches in whole, or in part, and lodges into a pulmonary artery. DVT can be clinically further subdivided according to: (1) its anatomic localization (proximal, if localized in the veins extending cephalad from where the calf veins (peroneal, anterior, and posterior tibial veins) join the popliteal vein (the trifurcation), or distal, if it is confined to the calf veins), and (2) whether it is symptomatic or not. As will be discussed later in this article, proximal and symptomatic DVT are more clinically relevant than distal and asymptomatic DVT.

It has been estimated that up to 50% of the patients with a symptomatic proximal DVT will have signs suggestive of PE on lung scans without any suggestive clinical symptoms.[1] Symptomatic VTE is usually treated with anticoagulant drugs because of its high mortality if untreated. The clinical relevance of symptomatic DVT or PE is highlighted by the fact that 50% of patients with an untreated symptomatic proximal DVT will experience a symptomatic PE within 3 months and around 10% of patients with a symptomatic PE will die shortly after onset.[2] It is therefore accepted that all patients with a PE or a symptomatic

[a] Department of Medicine, University of Western Ontario, 800 Commissioners Road, E PO Box 5010 Room A2-401, London, ON N6A 5W9, Canada
[b] Department of Oncology, University of Western Ontario, 800 Commissioners Road, E PO Box 5010 Room A2-401, London, ON N6A 5W9, Canada
[c] London Health Sciences Centre, Victoria Hospital, 800 Commissioners Road, E PO Box 5010 Room A2-401, London, ON N6A 5W9, Canada
[d] Department of Medicine, University of Ottawa, 501 Smyth Road Room 1812-E Box 201, Ottawa, ON K1H 8L6, Canada
[e] Department of Epidemiology and Community Medicine, University of Ottawa, 501 Smyth Road Room 1812-E Box 201, Ottawa, ON K1H 8L6, Canada
[f] Department of Obstetrics and Gynecology, University of Ottawa, 501 Smyth Road Room 1812-E Box 201, Ottawa, ON K1H 8L6, Canada
[g] Clinical Epidemiology Program, Ottawa Health Research Institute, 501 Smyth Road Room 1812-E Box 201, Ottawa, ON K1H 8L6, Canada
* Corresponding author. Ottawa Health Research Institute, Clinical Epedimiology Program, 501 Smyth Rd, Rm 1812-E Box 201, Ottawa, ON K1H 8L6 Canada.
E-mail address: mrodger@ohri.ca (M.A. Rodger).

Orthop Clin N Am 40 (2009) 427–436
doi:10.1016/j.ocl.2009.02.005

proximal DVT require treatment with the aim of preventing a recurrence.

The management of patients with an isolated distal DVT is controversial. This controversy arises from several facts. Firstly, thromboses occurring in association with surgery usually start in the veins of the calf; however, approximately one half will resolve spontaneously within 72 hours.[2] Secondly, only about one fifth to one sixth of the patients with a symptomatic distal DVT will experience an extension of a calf clot into the proximal veins.[3,4] Thirdly, although the risk of proximal extension in asymptomatic patients is likely lower, it remains unknown. Finally, the risk of PE is greatly increased when the thrombus extends into the proximal veins, but not if the clot remains confined to the calf.[3,4] For these reasons, the usual practice in North America is to treat patients with proximal DVT or PE and to perform serial ultrasounds in patients with isolated calf thromboses, and only treat those patients in whom the serial ultrasounds demonstrate an extension into the proximal veins.[5]

RISK OF VENOUS THROMBOEMBOLISM AFTER MAJOR ORTHOPEDIC SURGERY

Since the mid 1960s it has been reported that major orthopedic surgery, including total-hip replacement (THR) and total-knee replacement, leads to a high risk for developing venous thromboembolism. Since surgical practice and postoperative care have substantially changed in the last 40 years as a result of improved knowledge on pathophysiology, kinematics and materials science, it is likely that such changes have impacted on the prevalence of VTE. Some of the most relevant changes likely influencing the risk of VTE are (1) early postoperative ambulation and rehabilitation; (2) preoperative autologous blood donation; (3) hypotensive epidural anesthesia with epinephrine infusion; (4) shorter surgical times, minimizing femoral vein occlusion and blood loss during surgery; (5) pneumatic

compression and patient mobilization with foot exercises immediately after surgery. More recent studies have reported that without the use of prophylaxis following THR the prevalence of venographic VTE might be as high as 93% and that fatal pulmonary embolism may develop in up to 2% of patients.[6] **Table 1** summarizes the prevalence of VTE in patients undergoing major orthopedic surgery and not receiving prophylaxis reported in randomized trials published after 1980. In a retrospective cohort study conducted in the early 1990s of 1162 subjects with THR, who did not receive prophylaxis, Warwick and colleagues[7] demonstrated an in-hospital fatal PE rate of 0.3% (95% CI 0.05%–0.75%), a confirmed symptomatic PE rate of 0.7% (95% CI 0.3%–1.5%) and a confirmed symptomatic DVT rate of 1.0% (95% CI-0.4%–1.7%). Given that the venographic DVT rate in subjects with THR not receiving prophylaxis is up to 57%, of which up to 36% are proximal, it is clear that the large majority of venographic thrombi (even proximal ones) do not lead to symptomatic events[8,9]; furthermore, most asymptomatic thrombi do not appear to lead to postphlebitic syndrome.[10] Nonetheless, a rate of in-hospital symptomatic events occurring in up to 2% of patients undergoing an elective procedure is high enough to warrant prophylaxis.

The risk of developing postoperative VTE extends at least up to 35 days after the surgery and probably longer.[11] A large epidemiologic study suggested that even after the adoption of widespread prophylaxis the incidence of symptomatic VTE after major orthopedic surgery might be as high as 2.8% of patients at 91 days and that up to 76% of VTE events are diagnosed after hospital discharge.[11] In patients undergoing THR the risk of symptomatic VTE (DVT or PE) 30 to 42 days after hospital discharge is 3.0% to 4.0%,[7,11,12] and the risk of fatal PE is estimated to be 0.34% to 1.0% over 90 days in modern cohort studies.[7] Although this is a significant risk, the optimal strategy to reduce it is uncertain.

Table 1
Prevalence of venous thromboembolism after major orthopedic surgery in subjects receiving placebo included in trials published between 1980 and 2004

Procedure	Proximal DVT + PE (%)	Proximal and Distal DVT + PE (%)	Symptomatic VTE[a] (%)
Total-hip replacement	7.4–57.1	22.0–92.9	1.0–6.0
Total- knee replacement	5.9–20.4	58.7–70.6	29.4

[a] Includes symptomatic DVT and PE, and deaths in which PE could not be excluded as the cause.
Data from Refs.[47–55]

PROPHYLAXIS FOR VENOUS THROMBOEMBOLISM

Measures to prevent VTE after total joint replacement are almost universally used and probably the most widely disseminated guidelines are those proposed by the American College of Chest Physicians (ACCP). The current ACCP guidelines recommend administering prophylaxis for at least 10 days and up to 28 to 35 days for patients undergoing THR.[6] These recommendations have been made based on the best high quality available evidence and they are considered to be strong (ie, ACCP Grade 1A, meaning that they are derived from well-conducted, randomized clinical trials with consistent results, and that there is a high level of certainty that benefits do, or do not, outweigh risks). The recommended agents for prophylaxis include different anticoagulant drugs, such as low molecular weight heparin (eg, ardeparin, dalteparin, enoxaparin, nadroparin, reviparin and tinzaparin), vitamin-K antagonists and fondaparinux. However, other agents are, or have been, used or evaluated for this indication including aspirin, unfractionated heparin (UFH), ximelagatran, dextran, hirudins, danaparoid, dabigatran and argatroban, and others are currently under investigation, such as apixiban or rivaroxaban.

VENOUS THROMBOEMBOLISM PROPHYLAXIS AND BLEEDING COMPLICATIONS

Although undoubtedly beneficial, anticoagulant therapy is not free from complications, the most frequent of which is hemorrhage. Up to 17% of patients included in VTE treatment studies will experience a major bleeding episode during the first 3 months of treatment[13] and it has been estimated that the case-fatality rate of major bleeding episodes is greater than 13%.[14] Higher intensity of anticoagulation, longer duration of treatment, and individual characteristics of the patient, such as comorbidity or concomitant medication, influence the risk of bleeding.[13] The definition of major bleeding has varied among studies, complicating the evaluation of bleeding risks associated with the use of anticoagulants, and, only recently, has a standard definition been proposed.[15] The International Society on Thrombosis and Haemostasis proposed that a bleeding episode be considered as major if it was fatal, involved a critical organ, resulted in a significant decrease in hemoglobin, or resulted in transfusion of two units of red cells. A limitation of this definition is that it was proposed for nonsurgical patients, and since recent surgery is a risk factor for bleeding, especially if associated with other risk factors, its use in surgical population might not be adequate.

ASSESSING THE EVIDENCE FOR VENOUS THROMBOEMBOLIC DISEASE PROPHYLAXIS AFTER TOTAL-HIP REPLACEMENT
Validity of Efficacy Outcome Measures

Data on absolute risk of DVT posthip arthroplasty is often misinterpreted/misrepresented in studies using venographic efficacy outcomes (ie, a thrombosis demonstrated by mandatory venography irrespectively from its anatomic location, symptom occurrence, or clinical presentation). Although venographic outcomes appear to be correlated to symptomatic VTE this remains controversial since most asymptomatic distal DVT do not evolve to symptomatic DVT and do not lead to post-thrombotic syndrome. In other words, an absolute risk of DVT of 20% in a study using venographic outcomes may seem impressive, but it only translates into an absolute risk of symptomatic VTE of about 4%.[12] However, relying on symptomatic events is often impractical when planning a randomized trial evaluating VTE prophylaxis after a surgical procedure. The reasons are twofold. Firstly, symptoms are difficult to standardize due to their subjective nature, and they might be difficult to assess if the surgical procedure involves the lower limbs, which is the case in orthopedic surgery. Secondly, because symptomatic events are relatively infrequent after surgery, to demonstrate relevant risk reductions, large sample sizes would be required with the subsequent increase in research costs. For these reasons, surrogate endpoints have been sought and used as measures of efficacy in studies evaluating prophylaxis after surgical procedures. Compression ultrasound has been used as a screening technique after surgical procedures with poor results as can be judged from its poor interobserver agreement and low sensitivity.[16] Therefore, the usual endpoint in surgical trials is venography because it is a standard radiological technique with a good interobserver agreement that allows objective comparisons and central blinded adjudication of outcomes.[17–20]

The use of venographic endpoints in VTE prophylaxis studies of patients undergoing surgery is still a matter of debate. Some authors argue that venographic DVT is a valid surrogate,[12,20,21] and this surrogate has been widely adopted in clinical trials evaluating VTE prophylaxis in patients undergoing surgery. However, there are several potential concerns regarding the use of surrogate endpoints. An appropriate surrogate endpoint needs biologic plausibility, demonstration of its prognostic value for the clinical outcome, and evidence that treatment effects on the surrogate correspond to effects on the clinical outcome.[22] Despite the arguments suggesting that a reduction in venographic thrombosis parallels a reduction in symptomatic events,[12,20,21] the aforementioned conditions have not been convincingly demonstrated in studies evaluating VTE prophylaxis after orthopedic surgery. This is because the natural history of asymptomatic venographically demonstrated DVT is not known, since many clinicians find it difficult not to treat these patients. The uncertain clinical significance of isolated distal DVT complicates the interpretation of VTE prophylaxis studies relying on venographic endpoints because of the high proportion of thromboses confined to the calf that is detected by this technique. A particularly worrisome aspect of venographic endpoints is that despite a good interobserver reliability and standardized diagnostic criteria, there is substantial variation in the event rates between adjudicating centers,[21] which could be the result of systematic differences in the evaluation of the relevance of the venographic findings derived from different clinical schools.

Sample Size and Minimally Clinically Important Difference

A potential caveat of thromboprophylaxis literature is the abundance of small studies that are actually underpowered and misinterpreted as demonstrating equivalence between different strategies. The first step in the design of a methodologically sound study is to establish a minimal difference that is clinically important to detect, called the minimal clinically important difference (MCID). In thrombosis prevention research, commonly used MCID values include a 2% absolute reduction in symptomatic proximal DVT, a 1% absolute reduction in symptomatic PE, a 0.1% absolute reduction in fatal PE, and a 1% reduction in major bleeds. Therefore, MCID determines the sample size necessary for the study to be representative. For example, a study designed to detect a reduction of symptomatic proximal DVT from 6% to 4% would require more than 1800 subjects per group to have 80% power (the minimum power). Similarly, to detect a reduction in major bleeding events from 2% to 1% a study would require over 2300 subjects per group. Therefore, it is easy to appreciate that many of the available studies might be methodologically flawed and their validity should be questioned.

CONTROVERSIES FOR IN-HOSPITAL PROPHYLAXIS FOR VENOUS THROMBOEMBOLIC DISEASE AFTER TOTAL-HIP REPLACEMENT
In-hospital Venous Thromboembolic Disease Prophylaxis

Low molecular weight heparin versus warfarin
Colwell and coworkers demonstrated a significantly lower rate of symptomatic VTE in THR patients with low molecular weight heparin (LMWH; enoxaparin 30 mg sc twice a day) (0.3%) than adjusted dose warfarin (1.1%).[23] There were more major bleeds in the LMWH group (1.2%) than in the warfarin group (0.5%) and although this difference did not reach statistical significance it was very close ($P = .055$). Similarly, Hull and colleagues[24] have shown a reduction in proximal DVT with LMWH, dalteparin starting either 2 hours before or 4 or more hours after surgery, (0.8%) compared with adjusted dose warfarin (3.0%); although the subgroup starting the LMWH postoperatively did not have a statistically significant reduction in symptomatic events. The preoperative dose subgroup (but not the postoperative one) had significantly more major bleeds than the warfarin arm (8.9% versus 4.5%; $P = .01$).

Fondaparinux versus low molecular weight heparin
Turpie and colleagues[25] have shown in a meta-analysis that fondaparinux in major orthopedic surgery prophylaxis is superior to enoxaparin in preventing proximal DVT (symptomatic and asymptomatic), but not symptomatic VTE. However, there was a 1% increase in major bleeds. In these studies, postoperative enoxaparin was started 12 to 24 hours after surgery, yet fondaparinux was started 6 hours postoperatively. This raises the possibility that superiority was observed because of the different timing of anticoagulation rather than there being true differences in efficacy between fondaparinux and enoxaparin.

Timing of initiation of anticoagulant prophylaxis
Hull and colleagues[26] conducted a systematic review examining efficacy and safety of different timings of initiation of LMWH. The authors concluded that starting at 6 to 8 hours postoperatively at half the usual daily dose was more effective than the next day or 12 hours preoperative initiation of LMWH, and safer than immediate (2 hours) preoperative administration. However, Strebel and colleagues[8] performed a systematic review examining preoperative (12 hours or more before surgery), perioperative (within 12 hours before or after surgery) and postoperative (greater than 12 hours after surgery) LMWH initiation and

concluded that while perioperative regimens appeared to result in lower venographic DVT rates, they were associated with more major bleeding events. Furthermore, there is evidence suggesting that this is also true for fondaparinux.[27] The studies defined timings differently, but they suggest that closer proximity to surgery dosing is more effective and seems to be associated with higher bleeding rates. It is not known whether the increase in bleeding observed with closer proximity to surgery dosing holds for both pre- and postoperative close proximity dosing, but given the concern of epidural hematomas, immediate preoperative dosing is less commonly used in North America. Large randomized trials directly comparing different timing of initial prophylaxis administration are required to answer this question directly and definitively.

Are low molecular weight heparins interchangeable?

Only one trial has directly compared two LMWHs.[28] This study was underpowered to detect clinically meaningful differences, but showed no difference in venographic thrombi. A DVT treatment study comparing two LMWHs (dalteparin versus tinzaparin) showed no difference in efficacy or safety.[29] It is doubtful that an adequately-powered, randomized trial will ever be conducted to establish clinical equivalence between different LMWH preparations in VTE prophylaxis after THR, but based on the pharmacologic and scant clinical data available, this is likely the case.

Aspirin (ASA)

The PEP trial has created much discussion, but unfortunately raises more questions than answers about the role of aspirin in VTE prophyalxis after hip arthroplasty.[30] This study examined 160 mg of aspirin (ASA) started preoperatively and continued for 35 days postoperativley in subjects undergoing hip-fracture surgery, hip arthroplasty and knee arthroplasty. Objectively proven and adjudicated symptomatic venous thromboembolic events up to the day of hospital discharge were collected. While the study demonstrated a statistically significant reduction in VTE in 13,356 subjects with hip fracture, from 2.5% to 1.6%, there was an increase in transfused bleeding episodes of 0.6%. No statistically significant reduction was observed in 2648 subjects undergoing hip or knee arthroplasty with 1.1% experiencing symptomatic VTE in the ASA group compared with 1.4% in the placebo group. Many subjects also got other forms of prophylaxis (over 40%). Previous meta-analysis of venographic studies did not demonstrate a reduction in DVT and biologic data demonstrate that ASA does not importantly reduce thrombin activity.[31,32] In summary, ASA should not be used alone for antithrombotic prophylaxis after total-hip arthroplasty.

Postdischarge Prophylaxis

The risk of developing postoperative VTE extends at least up to 35 days after the surgery and probably longer.[33] A large epidemiologic study suggested that even after the adoption of widespread prophylaxis, the incidence of VTE after major orthopedic surgery might be as high as 2.8% of subjects at 91 days, and that up to 76% of VTE events are diagnosed after hospital discharge.[11] However, in randomized studies evaluating thromboprophylaxis after major orthopedic surgery and reporting a follow-up between 42 and 180 days, the occurrence of late events (ie, those occurring after completing an initial course of prophylaxis of less than 15 days of duration) was not exceedingly common (**Table 2**), in spite of which several randomized trials have shown that extended-duration anticoagulation reduces the risk of venographic and symptomatic VTE after

Table 2
Prevalence of venous thromboembolic events occurring up to 180 days after completing a course of short-term anticoagulant prophylaxis (› 15 days) reported in studies evaluating subjects undergoing major orthopedic surgery

Drug	Symptomatic DVT/PE (%)	Fatal Pulmonary Embolism (%)
Ximelagatran	0.26–1.54	0–0.77
LMW	0–3.1	0–0.67
UFH	0–2.68	0–0.67
Warfarin	0–1.47	0–0.13
Fondaparinux	0.62–1.69	0–0.72

Data from Refs.[23,49,51,56–76]

major orthopedic surgery[24,33–38] although one study did not find a significant reduction.[39] On the other hand, it has been argued that because of the low frequency of symptomatic events extended prophylaxis is not required.[7]

Low molecular weight heparin

Eikelboom conducted a meta-analysis examining postdischarge prophylaxis with LMWH after THR and demonstrated a reduction in symptomatic venous thromboembolism from 4.3% to 1.4% with LMWH.[12] The number needed to treat was 34. Enoxaparin (40 mg/day) and dalteparin (5000 U/day) were the most common regimens used. Although current recommendations suggest that patients should receive extended prophylaxis after THR[6] cost-effectiveness analyses are required. Patient preferences and risk stratification (eg, very obese patients, very immobilized patients, patients with thrombophilia or previous thrombosis) may be useful in making individual patient decisions about use of extended LMWH prophylaxis.

Vitamin-K antagonists

Prandoni and colleagues[40] conducted a randomized controlled trial examining continuing warfarin (for 4 weeks) versus discontinuing warfarin at the time of discharge after THR. All subjects had clinical and bilateral leg ultrasound follow-up at discharge and 1, 2, and 4 weeks later. There were statistically fewer recurrences in the warfarin arm (0.5%, 1/184) than in the no warfarin arm (5.1%) at 4 weeks, but not at 3 months. Major bleeding occurred in 0.5% of subjects on warfarin. Once again, cost effectiveness analyses are required. Again, patient preferences and risk stratification may be useful in making individual patient decisions about the use of extended warfarin prophylaxis.

Aspirin

ASA prophylaxis could be considered in patients who are not deemed to be at sufficient risk to warrant thromboprophylaxis with LMWH or warfarin. As outlined earlier in this article, primary evidence is not available to demonstrate a benefit, (although the hip-fracture data is compelling); given the little risk, inconvenience, and cost, the downsides are few. Randomized, controlled trials of postdischarge prophylaxis with ASA in large populations are ongoing.

NEW ANTICOAGULANT DRUGS

Because of the narrow therapeutic window of vitamin-K antagonists and the inconvenience of the parenteral route of administration of LMWH

and fondaparinux recently there have been considerable advances in the development of new anticoagulant drugs that can be easily administered, have an acceptable safety profile, and have a steady predictable response on the coagulation system, thus avoiding the need of frequent monitoring. Two new pharmacologic classes of agents, the direct thrombin inhibitors and the direct inhibitors of the activated coagulation factor X (anti-Xa), have recently been developed. Their mechanism of action may give these drugs some potential advantages over warfarin and LMWHs. Since thrombin is involved in many inflammatory reactions, direct thrombin inhibitors might limit inflammation in sites where a thrombus has developed. Some of these drugs inhibit the thrombin-mediated platelet activation process, thus yielding a theoretical advantage in patients with conditions such as coronary artery disease and possibly stroke. Because of these advantages, several agents have been studied for thromboprophylaxis after orthopedic surgery.

Oral Direct Thrombin Inhibitors

The first agent to be developed in this class was ximelagatran, a prodrug of the active form melagatran. Its mechanism of action involves a direct inhibition of the active site of thrombin in either its circulating or clot-bound forms, thus preventing the extension of a previously formed clot. Initial studies showed that this drug was efficacious and safe for VTE prophylaxis after orthopedic surgery; however, a meta-analysis showed that although in patients with THR the use of ximelagatran resulted in less VTE events compared with LMWH, it was also associated with a 3.33-fold increase in major bleeding.[41] Furthermore, after initial approval in Europe, unforeseen serious hepatic toxicity resulted in the drug being withdrawn from the market by the manufacturer. In spite of this, a related compound, dabigatran etexilate has been recently approved for VTE prophylaxis after orthopedic surgery in Canada and other countries. This drug has been proven to be at least equivalent to enoxaparin in large randomized trials and apparently is not associated with liver toxicity.[42,43]

Oral Direct Anti-Xa Inhibitors

Currently, there are two drugs within this class in clinical development. The first drug, apixiban, has been tested in subjects undergoing total-knee arthroplasty in a large phase II randomized trial with promising results.[44] Studies in THR are under development. The second drug is rivaroxaban which has been recently approved for VTE prophylaxis after major orthopedic surgery in Canada and elsewhere. Phase III studies have suggested that this agent is likely more effective than LMWH for preventing VTE after THR with a safety profile similar to LMWH.[45,46] Further studies are ongoing in this and other populations.

SUMMARY

Venous thromboembolic disease continues to be a serious complication of total-hip arthroplasty. The use of anticoagulant drugs for preventing this complication has repeatedly been proven to be useful. More aggressive anticoagulant agents, or schedules, have been shown to result in less thrombotic episodes; however they also seem to be associated with higher bleeding risks. The current evidence-based recommendations are to administer prophylaxis with warfarin, LMWH, or fondaparinux, for at least 10, and up to 35, days after surgery. Special attention should be paid to patients at high risk for both thrombosis and bleeding to choose the most appropriate prophylactic method, and ultimately, a judicious individual consideration by the treating clinician should guide the final decision. The advent of new anticoagulant drugs is a very active area of research and several agents have shown promising results. Finally, several issues such as optimal dose, drug interchangeability, timing, and validity of surrogate outcomes remain uncertain.

REFERENCES

1. Huisman MV, Buller HR, Ten Cate JW, et al. Unexpected high prevalence of silent pulmonary embolism in patients with deep venous thrombosis. Chest 1989;95(3):498–502.
2. Kearon C. Natural history of venous thromboembolism. Circulation 2003;107(23 Suppl 1):I-22–30.
3. Masuda EM, Kessler DM, Kistner RL, et al. The natural history of calf vein thrombosis: lysis of thrombi and development of reflux. J Vasc Surg 1998;28(1):67–73.
4. Philbrick JT, Becker DM. Calf deep venous thrombosis. A wolf in sheep's clothing? Arch Intern Med 1988;148(10):2131–8.
5. Scarvelis D, Wells PS. Diagnosis and treatment of deep-vein thrombosis. CMAJ 2006;175(9):1087–92.
6. Geerts WH, Bergqvist D, Pineo GF, et al. Prevention of venous thromboembolism: American college of chest physicians evidence-based clinical practice guidelines. 8th edition. Chest 2008;133(Suppl 6):381S–453S.
7. Warwick D, Williams MH, Bannister GC. Death and thromboembolic disease after total hip replacement.

A series of 1162 cases with no routine chemical prophylaxis. J Bone Joint Surg Br 1995;77-B(1):6–10.
8. Strebel N, Prins M, Agnelli G, et al. Preoperative or postoperative start of prophylaxis for venous thromboembolism with low-molecular-weight heparin in elective hip surgery? Arch Intern Med 2002; 162(13):1451–6.
9. Hirsh J, Dalen J, Guyatt G. The sixth (2000) ACCP guidelines for antithrombotic therapy for prevention and treatment of thrombosis. American College of Chest Physicians. Chest 2001;119(Suppl 1):1S–2S.
10. Ginsberg JS, Turkstra F, Buller HR, et al. Postthrombotic syndrome after hip or knee arthroplasty: a cross-sectional study. Arch Intern Med 2000; 160(5):669–72.
11. White RH, Romano PS, Zhou H, et al. Incidence and time course of thromboembolic outcomes following total hip or knee arthroplasty. Arch Intern Med 1998;158(14):1525–31.
12. Eikelboom JW, Quinlan DJ, Douketis JD. Extended-duration prophylaxis against venous thromboembolism after total hip or knee replacement: a meta-analysis of the randomised trials. Lancet 2001;358(9275):9–15.
13. Schulman S, Beyth RJ, Kearon C, et al. Hemorrhagic complications of anticoagulant and thrombolytic treatment: American College of Chest Physicians Evidence-Based Clinical Practice Guidelines. 8th edition. Chest 2008;133(Suppl 6):257S–98S.
14. Linkins LA, Choi PT, Douketis JD. Clinical impact of bleeding in patients taking oral anticoagulant therapy for venous thromboembolism: a meta-analysis. Ann Intern Med 2003;139(11):893–900.
15. Schulman S, Kearon C. Definition of major bleeding in clinical investigations of antihemostatic medicinal products in non-surgical patients. J Thromb Haemost 2005;3(4):692–4.
16. Schellong SM, Beyer J, Kakkar AK, et al. Ultrasound screening for asymptomatic deep vein thrombosis after major orthopaedic surgery: the VENUS study. J Thromb Haemost 2007;5(7):1431–7.
17. Rabinov K, Paulin S. Roentgen diagnosis of venous thrombosis in the leg. Arch Surg 1972;104(2):134–44.
18. Kalodiki E, Nicolaides AN, Al-Kutoubi A, et al. How "gold" is the standard? Interobservers' variation on venograms. Int Angiol 1998;17(2):83–8.
19. Kalebo P, Ekman S, Lindbratt S, et al. Percentage of inadequate phlebograms and observer agreement in thromboprophylactic multicenter trials using standardized methodology and central assessment. Thromb Haemost 1996;76(6):893–6.
20. Segers AEM, Prins MH, Lensing AWA, et al. Is contrast venography a valid surrogate outcome measure in venous thromboembolism prevention studies? J Thromb Haemost 2005;3(5):1099–102.
21. Quinlan DJ, Eikelboom JW, Dahl OE, et al. Association between asymptomatic deep-vein thrombosis

detected by venography and symptomatic venous thromboembolism in patients undergoing elective hip or knee surgery. J Thromb Haemost 2007;5(7): 1438–43.

22. ICH Harmonised Tripartite Guideline. Statistical Principles for Clinical Trials. International Conference on Harmonisation of Technical Requirements for Registration of Pharmaceuticals for Human Use. Report E9; 1998. Available at: http://www.ich.org/LOB/media/MEDIA485.pdf. Accessed June 5, 2009.

23. Colwell CW Jr, Collis DK, Paulson R, et al. Comparison of enoxaparin and warfarin for the prevention of venous thromboembolic disease after total hip arthroplasty. Evaluation during hospitalization and three months after discharge. J Bone Joint Surg Am 1999;81(7):932–40.

24. Hull RD, Pineo GF, Francis C, et al. Low-molecular-weight heparin prophylaxis using dalteparin extended out-of-hospital vs in-hospital warfarin/out-of-hospital placebo in hip arthroplasty patients: a double-blind, randomized comparison. North American Fragmin Trial Investigators. Arch Intern Med 2000;160(14):2208–15 2199–2207.

25. Turpie AGG, Bauer KA, Eriksson BI, et al. for the Steering Committees of the Pentasaccharide Orthopedic Prophylaxis Studies. Fondaparinux vs enoxaparin for the prevention of venous thromboembolism in major orthopedic surgery: a meta-analysis of 4 randomized double-blind studies. Arch Intern Med 2002;162(16):1833–40.

26. Hull RD, Pineo GF, Stein PD, et al. Timing of initial administration of low-molecular-weight heparin prophylaxis against deep vein thrombosis in patients following elective hip arthroplasty. A systematic review. Arch Intern Med 2001;161:1952–60.

27. Turpie AGG, Bauer KA, Eriksson BI, et al. Efficacy and safety of fondaparinux in major orthopedic surgery according to the timing of its first administration. Thromb Haemost 2003;90:364–6.

28. Planes A, Samama MM, Lensing AW, et al. Prevention of deep vein thrombosis after hip replacement–comparison between two low-molecular heparins, tinzaparin and enoxaparin. Thromb Haemost 1999;81(1):22–5.

29. Wells PS, Anderson DR, Rodger MA, et al. A randomized trial comparing 2 low-molecular-weight heparins for the outpatient treatment of deep vein thrombosis and pulmonary embolism. Arch Intern Med 2005;165(7):733–8.

30. Pulmonary Embolism Prevention (PEP) Trial Collaborative Group. Prevention of pulmonary embolism and deep vein thrombosis with low dose aspirin: pulmonary embolism prevention (PEP) trial. Lancet 2000;355(9212):1295–302.

31. Imperiale TF, Speroff T. A meta-analysis of methods to prevent venous thromboembolism following total hip replacement. JAMA 1994;271(22):1780–5.

32. Kessels H, Beguin S, Andree H, et al. Measurement of thrombin generation in whole blood–the effect of heparin and aspirin. Thromb Haemost 1994;72(1): 78–83.

33. Planes A, Vochelle N, Darmon JY, et al. Risk of deep-venous thrombosis after hospital discharge in patients having undergone total hip replacement: double-blind randomised comparison of enoxaparin versus placebo. Lancet 1996;48(9022):224–8.

34. Comp PC, Spiro TE, Friedman RJ, et al. Prolonged enoxaparin therapy to prevent venous thromboembolism after primary hip or knee replacement. Enoxaparin Clinical Trial Group. J Bone Joint Surg Am 2001;83(3):336–45.

35. Lassen MR, Borris LC, Anderson BS, et al. Efficacy and safety of prolonged thromboprophylaxis with a low molecular weight heparin (dalteparin) after total hip arthroplasty–the Danish Prolonged Prophylaxis (DaPP) Study. Thromb Res 1998;89(6):281–7.

36. Dahl OE, Andreassen G, Aspelin T, et al. Prolonged thromboprophylaxis following hip replacement surgery–results of a double-blind, prospective, randomised, placebo-controlled study with dalteparin (Fragmin). Thromb Haemost 1997;77(1):26–31.

37. Bergqvist D, Benoni G, Bjorgell O, et al. Low-molecular-weight heparin (enoxaparin) as prophylaxis against venous thromboembolism after total hip replacement. N Engl J Med 1996;335(10):696–700.

38. Hull RD, Pineo GF, Stein PD, et al. Extended out-of-hospital low-molecular-weight heparin prophylaxis against deep venous thrombosis in patients after elective hip arthroplasty: a systematic review. Ann Intern Med 2001;135(10):858–69.

39. Heit JA, Elliott CG, Trowbridge AA, et al. Ardeparin sodium for extended out-of-hospital prophylaxis against venous thromboembolism after total hip or knee replacement. A randomized, double-blind, placebo-controlled trial. Ann Intern Med 2000; 132(11):853–61.

40. Prandoni P, Bruchi O, Sabbion P, et al. Prolonged thromboprophylaxis with oral anticoagulants after total hip arthroplasty: a prospective controlled randomized study. Arch Intern Med 2002;162(17):1966–71.

41. Lazo-Langner A, Rodger MA, Wells PS. Lessons from ximelagatran. Issues for future studies evaluating new oral direct thrombin inhibitors for venous thromboembolism prophylaxis in orthopedic surgery. Clin Appl Thromb Hemost, in press.

42. Eriksson BI, Dahl OE, Buller HR, et al. A new oral direct thrombin inhibitor, dabigatran etexilate, compared with enoxaparin for prevention of thromboembolic events following total hip or knee replacement: the BISTRO II randomized trial. J Thromb Haemost 2005;3(1):103–11.

43. Eriksson BI, Dahl OE, Ahnfelt L, et al. Dose escalating safety study of a new oral direct thrombin inhibitor, dabigatran etexilate, in patients undergoing total hip

replacement: BISTRO I. J Thromb Haemost 2004; 2(9):1573–80.

44. Lassen MR, Davidson BL, Gallus A, et al. The efficacy and safety of apixaban, an oral, direct factor Xa inhibitor, as thromboprophylaxis in patients following total knee replacement. J Thromb Haemost 2007;5(12):2368–75.

45. Eriksson BI, Borris LC, Friedman RJ, et al. Rivaroxaban versus enoxaparin for thromboprophylaxis after hip arthroplasty. N Engl J Med 2008;358(26):2765–75.

46. Fisher WD, Eriksson BI, Bauer KA, et al. Rivaroxaban for thromboprophylaxis after orthopaedic surgery: pooled analysis of two studies. Thromb Haemost 2007;97(6):931–7.

47. Kalodiki EP, Hoppensteadt DA, Nicolaides AN, et al. Deep venous thrombosis prophylaxis with low molecular weight heparin and elastic compression in patients having total hip replacement. A randomised controlled trial. Int Angiol 1996;15(2):162–8.

48. Lassen MR, Borris LC, Christiansen HM, et al. Prevention of thromboembolism in 190 hip arthroplasties. Comparison of LMW heparin and placebo. Acta Orthop Scand 1991;62(1):33–8.

49. Leclerc JR, Geerts WH, Desjardins L, et al. Prevention of deep vein thrombosis after major knee surgery–a randomized, double-blind trial comparing a low molecular weight heparin fragment (enoxaparin) to placebo. Thromb Haemost 1992;67(4):417–23.

50. Levine MN, Gent M, Hirsh J, et al. Ardeparin (low-molecular-weight heparin) vs graduated compression stockings for the prevention of venous thromboembolism. A randomized trial in patients undergoing knee surgery. Arch Intern Med 1996; 156(8):851–6.

51. Torholm C, Broeng L, Jorgensen PS, et al. Thromboprophylaxis by low-molecular-weight heparin in elective hip surgery. A placebo controlled study. J Bone Joint Surg Br 1991;73(3):434–8.

52. Turpie AG, Levine MN, Hirsh J, et al. A randomized controlled trial of a low-molecular-weight heparin (enoxaparin) to prevent deep-vein thrombosis in patients undergoing elective hip surgery. N Eng J Med 1986;315(15):925–9.

53. Wang CJ, Wang JW, Weng LH, et al. Prevention of deep-vein thrombosis after total knee arthroplasty in Asian patients. Comparison of low-molecular-weight heparin and indomethacin. J Bone Joint Surg Am 2004;86(1):136–40.

54. Warwick D, Bannister GC, Glew D, et al. Perioperative low-molecular-weight heparin. Is it effective and safe. J Bone Joint Surg Br 1995;77(5):715–9.

55. Yoo MC, Kang CS, Kim YH, et al. A prospective randomized study on the use of nadroparin calcium in the prophylaxis of thromboembolism in Korean patients undergoing elective total hip replacement. Int Orthop 1997;21(6):399–402.

56. The TIFDED Study Group. Thromboprophylaxis in hip fracture surgery: a pilot study comparing danaparoid, enoxaparin and dalteparin. Haemostasis 1999;29(6):310–7.

57. Eriksson BI, Agnelli G, Cohen AT, et al. The direct thrombin inhibitor melagatran followed by oral ximelagatran compared with enoxaparin for the prevention of venous thromboembolism after total hip or knee replacement: the EXPRESS study. J Thromb Haemost 2003;1(12):2490–6.

58. Colwell CW Jr, Berkowitz SD, Davidson BL, et al. Comparison of ximelagatran, an oral direct thrombin inhibitor, with enoxaparin for the prevention of venous thromboembolism following total hip replacement. A randomized, double-blind study. J Thromb Haemost 2003;1(10):2119–30.

59. Navarro-Quilis A, Castellet E, Rocha E, et al. Bemiparin Study Group. Efficacy and safety of bemiparin compared with enoxaparin in the prevention of venous thromboembolism after total knee arthroplasty: a randomized, double-blind clinical trial. J Thromb Haemost 2003;1(3):425–32.

60. Eriksson BI, Agnelli G, Cohen AT, et al. Direct thrombin inhibitor melagatran followed by oral ximelagatran in comparison with enoxaparin for prevention of venous thromboembolism after total hip or knee replacement. Thromb Haemost 2003;89(2):288–96.

61. Eriksson BI, Bergqvist D, Kalebo P, et al. Ximelagatran and melagatran compared with dalteparin for prevention of venous thromboembolism after total hip or knee replacement: the METHRO II randomised trial. Lancet 2002;360(9344):1441–7.

62. Francis CW, Davidson BL, Berkowitz SD, et al. Ximelagatran versus warfarin for the prevention of venous thromboembolism after total knee arthroplasty. A randomized, double-blind trial. Ann Intern Med 2002;137(8):648–55.

63. Turpie AG, Bauer KA, Eriksson BI, et al. Study Steering Committee. Postoperative fondaparinux versus postoperative enoxaparin for prevention of venous thromboembolism after elective hip-replacement surgery: a randomised double-blind trial. Lancet 2002;359(9319):1721–6.

64. Lassen MR, Bauer KA, Eriksson BI, et al. European Pentasaccharide Elective Surgery Study (EPHESUS) Steering Committee. Postoperative fondaparinux versus preoperative enoxaparin for prevention of venous thromboembolism in elective hip-replacement surgery: a randomised double-blind comparison. Lancet 2002;359(9319):1715–20.

65. Eriksson BI, Bauer KA, Lassen MR, et al. Steering Committee of the Pentasaccharide in Hip-Fracture Surgery Study. Fondaparinux compared with enoxaparin for the prevention of venous thromboembolism after hip-fracture surgery. N Eng J Med 2001; 345(18):1298–304.

66. Heit JA, Colwell CW, Francis CW, et al. Comparison of the oral direct thrombin inhibitor ximelagatran with enoxaparin as prophylaxis against venous thromboembolism after total knee replacement: a phase 2 dose-finding study. Arch Intern Med 2001;161(18):2215–21.

67. Turpie AG, Gallus AS, Hoek JA, et al. A synthetic pentasaccharide for the prevention of deep-vein thrombosis after total hip replacement. N Eng J Med 2001;344(9):619–25.

68. Kakkar VV, Howes J, Sharma V, et al. A comparative double-blind, randomised trial of a new second generation LMWH (bemiparin) and UFH in the prevention of post-operative venous thromboembolism. The Bemiparin Assessment group. Thromb Haemost 2000;83(4):523–9.

69. Leclerc JR, Geerts WH, Desjardins L, et al. Prevention of venous thromboembolism after knee arthroplasty. A randomized, double-blind trial comparing enoxaparin with warfarin. Ann Intern Med 1996; 124(7):619–26.

70. Fauno P, Suomalainen O, Rehnberg V, et al. Prophylaxis for the prevention of venous thromboembolism after total knee arthroplasty. A comparison between unfractionated and low-molecular-weight heparin. J Bone Joint Surg Am 1994;76(12):1814–8.

71. Spiro TE, Johnson GJ, Christie MJ, et al. Efficacy and safety of enoxaparin to prevent deep venous thrombosis after hip replacement surgery. Enoxaparin Clinical Trial Group. Ann Intern Med 1994;121(2):81–9.

72. Hull R, Raskob G, Pineo G, et al. A comparison of subcutaneous low-molecular-weight heparin with warfarin sodium for prophylaxis against deep-vein thrombosis after hip or knee implantation. N Eng J Med 1993;329(19):1370–6.

73. The German Hip Arthroplasty Trial (GHAT) Group. Prevention of deep vein thrombosis with low molecular-weight heparin in patients undergoing total hip replacement. A randomized trial. Arch Orthop Trauma Surg 1992;111(2):110–20.

74. Leyvraz PF, Bachmann F, Hoek J, et al. Prevention of deep vein thrombosis after hip replacement: randomised comparison between unfractionated heparin and low molecular weight heparin. Br Med J 1991; 303(6802):543–8.

75. Colwell CW Jr, Berkowitz SD, Lieberman JR, et al. Oral direct thrombin inhibitor ximelagatran compared with warfarin for the prevention of venous thromboembolism after total knee arthroplasty. J Bone Joint Surg Am 2005;87(10):2169–77.

76. Bauer KA, Eriksson BI, Lassen MR, et al. The Steering Committee of the Pentasaccharide in Major Knee Surgery Study. Fondaparinux compared with enoxaparin for the prevention of venous thromboembolism after elective major knee surgery. N Eng J Med 2001;345(18):1305–10.

Index

Note: Page numbers of article titles are in **boldface** type.

Orthop Clin N Am 40 (2009) 437–440
doi:10.1016/S0030-5898(09)00051-0
0030-5898/09/$ – see front matter © 2009 Elsevier Inc. All rights reserved.

orthopedic.theclinics.com

Moving?

Make sure your subscription moves with you!

To notify us of your new address, find your **Clinics Account Number** (located on your mailing label above your name), and contact customer service at:

E-mail: elspcs@elsevier.com

800-654-2452 (subscribers in the U.S. & Canada)
314-453-7041 (subscribers outside of the U.S. & Canada)

Fax number: 314-523-5170

Elsevier Periodicals Customer Service
11830 Westline Industrial Drive
St. Louis, MO 63146

*To ensure uninterrupted delivery of your subscription, please notify us at least 4 weeks in advance of move.

Printed and bound by CPI Group (UK) Ltd, Croydon, CR0 4YY

03/10/2024

01040361-0012